Make Your Life Better

You will spend a third of your life in the "freedom third", the years after your formal retirement. We believe this freedom gives each of you a marvelous opportunity—the opportunity to release the unique person that is contained within you.

You have now reached a point in life that calls for an important decision. A life of wonder and beauty is possible for you.

We assume that you want to enjoy life, that you will live a long time, and that you want to design the last third of your life for fun and freedom. This is a book about living your dreams...

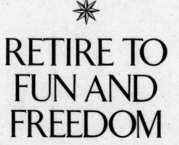

RETIRE TO FUN AND FREEDOM

RETIRE TO FUN AND FREEDOM

Louise McCants and Cavett Robert

A Warner Communications Company

Warner Books Edition
Copyright © 1988 by Louise McCants and Cavett Robert
All rights reserved.
This Warner Books edition is published by arrangement with the authors.
Warner Books, Inc., 666 Fifth Avenue, New York, NY 10103

 A Warner Communications Company

Printed in the United States of America
First Warner Books Printing: May 1990
10 9 8 7 6 5 4 3 2 1

Library of Congress Cataloging in Publication Data

McCants, Louise Spears.
    Retire to fun and freedom / by Louise McCants and Cavett Robert. —
Warner Books ed.
    p. cm.
    Reprint. Originally published: Kansas City, Mo. : Vive
Publications, 1988.
    ISBN 0-446-39139-5
    1. Retirement—United States—Psychological aspects. 2. Retirees—
United States—Life skills guides.   I. Robert, Cavett. II. Title.
HQ1063.2.U6M35   1990
306.3′8′0973—dc20   89-70545
                                                                                                     CIP

Cover design by Harold Nolan
Cover photograph by Four by Five/Superstock

ATTENTION: SCHOOLS AND CORPORATIONS

Warner books are available at quantity discounts with bulk purchase for educational, business, or sales promotional use. For information, please write to: Special Sales Department, Warner Books, 666 Fifth Avenue, New York, NY 10103.

ARE THERE WARNER BOOKS YOU WANT BUT CANNOT FIND IN YOUR LOCAL STORES?

You can get any **Warner Books** title in print. Simply send title and retail price, plus 50¢ per order and 50¢ per copy to cover mailing and handling costs for each book desired. New York State and California residents, add applicable sales tax. Enclose check or money order—no cash, please—to: **Warner Books, PO Box 690, New York, NY 10019.** Or send for our complete catalog of Warner Books.

ABOUT THE AUTHORS

Louise McCants

Louise McCants is an educator with many years of teaching experience and twenty years of administrative experience. A native of Appleton, Arkansas, she received B.S. and M.S. degrees in mathematics from Oklahoma State University, and a Ph.D. in adult education from The Ohio State University. She is nationally recognized as a consultant and speaker in adult and community college education. She is the author of *Womanchange! Choosing What's Best for You,* and has published extensively on women's issues. She designed and implemented a pre-retirement planning program which in 1986 was funded by the U.S. Department of Health and Human Services as a national model.

* * * * * *

Cavett Robert

Cavett Robert was born in Starkville, Mississippi. He received his B.A. degree from the University of Mississippi and a degree in law from Washington and Lee University, Virginia. His ability to add people knowledge to product knowledge has earned him the reputation of the number one speaker in America in the field of human engineering and motivation. He has received numerous awards: the coveted Golden Gavel Award given by Toastmasters International to the nation's outstanding speaker in the field of leadership and communication, the Speakers Hall of Fame Award, and the International Toastmasters Award. He is the author of the popular book, *The Cavett Robert Personal Development Course,* as well as several other books and over a dozen inspirational recordings.

His knowledge in sales and human relations is drawn

from a wide background of experience. A lawyer by profession, he has sold insurance and real estate, coordinated sales schools, and conducted courses for many of the nation's outstanding companies. He is the founder of the National Speakers Association and since his formal retirement eighteen years ago has addressed more than 3,500 audiences.

CONTENTS

I. PHILOSOPHY
   CHAPTER 1.
     HOW TO RETIRE TO FUN AND FREEDOM 12
   CHAPTER 2.
     THE TIME OF YOUR LIFE 20
   CHAPTER 3.
     BEYOND MATERIALISM 32
   CHAPTER 4.
     WHAT DOES YOUR FUTURE HOLD? 38

II. METHODS
   CHAPTER 5.
     DECIDE WHAT YOU REALLY WANT 48
   CHAPTER 6.
     MATCH YOUR TALENTS TO YOUR TASK 59
   CHAPTER 7.
     CHOOSE YOUR NEXT CAREER 68
   CHAPTER 8.
     REACH YOUR FULL POTENTIAL 80
   CHAPTER 9.
     FLOURISH IN ADVERSITY 89
   CHAPTER 10.
     FIND LIFE AFTER LAY-OFF 103
   CHAPTER 11.
     CHOOSE YOUR TASK 111
   CHAPTER 12.
     EXPAND YOUR HORIZONS 119

CHAPTER 13.
  PERSUADE OTHERS   127
CHAPTER 14.
  LIVE HARMONIOUSLY WITH OTHERS   136

III. THE REWARDS
  CHAPTER 15.
    TO ENJOY THE LIFE YOU HAVE EARNED   148
  CHAPTER 16.
    ADD LIFE TO YOUR YEARS   159
  CHAPTER 17.
    THE DIPLOMA—HAPPINESS   171

YOUR PERSONAL CHARTS
A. YOUR HAPPINESS CHART   TABLE I   49
B. YOUR LIST OF STRENGTHS TABLE II   52
C. YOUR TALENT TABLE   TABLE III   62
D. YOUR JOB ANALYSIS   TABLE IV,   65
                           PART A
                           TABLE IV,   65
                           PART B
E. YOUR PERSONAL DECISION TABLE   73
                           TABLE V
F. YOUR ENJOYMENT CHART   TABLE VI   152

RETIRE TO FUN AND FREEDOM

PREFACE

Americans are retiring earlier and living longer than ever before. This book is intended as their guide into new territory—the twenty or thirty years of freedom that most can expect after their first formal retirement.

One fourth of America's population, approximately sixty million people, are now 50 years old or older, and either retiring or thinking about it. With an average life expectancy at age 50 of another 26 years, many can confidently plan on spending one third of their lives in their freedom phase. This new longevity brings a new set of values.

The man who retired at age 65 at the turn of the last century measured his remaining life expectancy in months rather than in years. In our time, when the average person retires at 61, in excellent health, new values and new hopes have emerged.

For many people over 60, the prosperity made possible during the industrialized post World War II economy has led to financial security. Theirs is a luxurious position. Freed of the necessity to work for wages, those in this fortunate group are ready to resume the dreams of their youth. Many will turn to volunteer work as a way of repaying a personal debt to the blessings of democracy. The profits of their efforts will be measured through service.

Others, now in their fifties and shifted prematurely out of their jobs by the economic upheavals of the past decade, are in the position of having to retire and retread. Too young to stop working, and too old to be willing to begin again at the bottom of the pay scale, these people are wondering how best to begin the final career phase of their lives. They need to make money, but they want to enjoy life in the process.

This book is written for both groups. It is exuberantly and unabashedly motivational, for we believe the time is ripe for a nation of mature entrepreneurs. The secret of each success will be to match individual talents to the new opportunities of an information age.

The powerful economic and demographic forces propelling this country into the next century can be made to work to the advantage of retirees. The rush toward technology is revolutionizing the economy; unprecedented longevity is producing a concurrent sociological revolution. The productive use of the talents of retirees can establish a happy linkage between these two revolutions.

In this time of transition, the qualities needed for success are limited neither by sex nor by age. Success in the next decade will depend on knowledge, people skills, and entrepreneurial ability. The opportunities are everywhere.

The retiree who expects to live well into the next century will bring an impressive set of skills to his freedom years. The employment of the talents of these energetic and capable citizens may be the foundation of the restoration of the American dream. Our country's renaissance may be made possible by a mature and talented group which exists only in America—the sixty million people enjoying health and the good life in their freedom third!

I. PHILOSOPHY

CHAPTER I
HOW TO RETIRE TO FUN AND FREEDOM

"It is impossible to live pleasurably without living wisely, well, and justly, and it is impossible to live wisely, well, and justly without living pleasurably." Epicurus...300 B.C.

At last you have the chance to live your dreams. Do you still remember what they were? If you dusted off the dreams of your youth and the hopes of your middle years and compared them now with your expectations for your future, would there be any points in common? Many of us have kept the same elusive dreams. For many more, the dreams have changed for the better. A few may have forgotten how to dream at all.

This is a book about living your dreams. The authors assume that you want to enjoy life, that you will live a long time, and that you want to design the last third of your life to fun and freedom.

We are living in a time when the lifespan of American adults is cause for celebration. Four in five of us can expect to reach age 65. Of those who do, at least half will live to be 85. The number of us over age 85 will triple by the year 2025. There is a good chance that you will spend a third of your life in your freedom third, the years after your formal retirement.

We believe this freedom gives each of you a marvelous opportunity—the opportunity to release the unique person who is contained within you. The dictionary defines your special quality as sui generis: of its own kind; unique. So this is a description about the path to sui generis—the journey toward becoming your own special self. This is a book about enjoying life.

This book was not statistically researched so as to be representative of the entire population of retired persons. It is, in fact, the exact opposite. We have deliberately sought out and interviewed people who are having such a good time in their freedom phase that they believe it is the best time of their lives. These people are having fun. Some of them are making money. Others are not spending their time to make money at all, but are devoting their efforts to public service, of which the profits of their work are shared with the population in general.

We talked with people across the country, and found a pattern which we could trace in the lives of all who are truly enjoying their retirement years. Invariably, those in this fortunate situation have one trait in common. They have deliberately chosen to do what they most enjoy doing. They have made up their minds to enjoy life, and have designed a way of living that supports this choice.

These people come in all shapes and sizes and places. Some of them you will meet in later chapters. A retired university football coach is now a troubleshooter for one of the nation's leading senators; a farmer is now a music teacher; a former housewife became a highly popular politician; a general practitioner has retired from medicine to found his own furniture company; a social worker has been transformed into a raconteur, a leader of a jazz combo, and thoroughly happy man about town. We talked to a saleswoman turned hatcheck girl, a dean turned airport limo driver, a weapons systems expert turned community volunteer, and an eighty two year old orthodontist whose practice is growing so steadily that he has no intention of retiring.

All of these and hundreds more share a common bond—a spirit so vital that it transcends the boundaries of time. We talked to dozens of persons who retired from working for someone else and began their own businesses in closely related fields. We believe that no more fortuitous time for the small business can be found than the world of the next decade. The opportunities are everywhere. This book has been written to help you design your own opportunity.

If the years have shifted your sights along with your center of gravity, you may need to spend some time getting acquainted with yourself. The person who emerges in retirement from the constraining cloak of structured duty may be a comparative stranger. But this person is a fascinating stranger, and one you need to know. Your acquaintance with your own unique self is essential to your future happiness. Your retirement will contain neither fun nor freedom until you come to understand that most interesting of persons—yourself. Approach this person with confidence, and begin the study of the art and science of sui generis—of becoming the self you always had it in you to be. Advance to meet your potential.

To map a guide for another is an act of presumption. It presumes the merit of the path, the competence of the guide, and the interest of the pilgrim.

In this sense, the book you are about to read is a presumptuous act. Its justification becomes a matter of conscience for the authors. Our reasons for writing it are to be found in our own life experiences. While our paths through life have been separate, we are joined in a common philosophy and purpose. It is this philosophy and its accompanying strategies which we will describe in the chapters of this book. When we use stories from our own experiences to illustrate particular points, we will use our first names, Cavett and Louise, in the telling.

The sum of our ages now amounts to more than fourteen decades. Cavett has given his life to the law and to the field of human development. Louise has spent her years as a college teacher and administrator, and has designed and implemented a preretirement training center in a major midwestern city. We have long since lost count of the number of persons with whom we have enjoyed the privilege of counsel. What we have retained is a sure sense of an undergirding framework of life's laws.

This book represents our combined effort to distill our understanding of these rules of human development, and to translate for you what it takes to be happy in retirement. We claim no wisdom beyond that accessible to any other. Nor do we claim that our philosophies require special circumstances for development. Since one of us was born in Appleton, Arkansas, and the other in Starkville, Mississippi, it is evident that we are not speaking from the point of view of the rich and famous. But we do call frequently on the wisdom of others who have earned fame in our civilization, many of whom are quoted in the chapters to follow.

It is our hope that by allowing our minds to hold

converse with your own that you will be stimulated into designing your own preferred pathway through the freedom third of your life. We know that we have set an immense task for ourselves. William James spoke truly when he said, "The most immutable barrier in nature is between one man's thoughts and another's." It is a task we joyously attempt, for we believe that the retirement years can be lived with grace and with grit, with vigor and with virtue, with wisdom and with gladness, and that none of these negates the other.

There exists as yet no formal certification process which in itself will testify to the expertise of one who claims to be a professional in preretirement planning. Success in the retirement years is measured as much by state of mind as state of bank account, and more by state of health than either of these.

Most experts agree that there are three areas of major importance: physical health, mental health, and financial health. The authors will attempt to establish their credibility in the first two while asserting that the third follows. Louise hiked the peaks of Glacier National Park during the summer of her 59th year; her first book was published when she was 62. Cavett established a new career, defined a new profession, and established a new organization, the National Speakers Association, after he retired from the practice of law. Both of us can testify to the zest and happiness which evolve from living our dreams.

The rewards which you will find when you decide to live your own dreams will not be different from our rewards. We believe that success is living the kind of life you **want** to live on terms which enrich you and the world around you. This definition of success is within the reach of us all. The coin common to all is the coin of talent. While the forms of our talents differ, the method of exchange is universal: when we are true to our best selves, it then becomes impossible to be false to any man. The search for truth and the avoidance of false goals is the essence of your enjoyment of life.

This book is written for the person who desires to go beyond the average. You now have reached a point in life which calls for an important decision. Making choices is difficult at best, and immobilizing at worst. Most of us live our lives following conventional pathways, those which have been trodden smooth by the feet of the multitude. By definition, the ways of the multitude are the ways of mediocrity, the ways of the average. Choosing to take the less traveled path is not easy. Basic to the human condition is the reluctance to depart from the average established by the many. But it is impossible to please everyone and impossible to have everything.

Given these conditions, it seems reasonable that each should chose the path that leads to individual accomplishment, harnessing talents and temperament toward the rewards of success. This success is all the sweeter for having been programmed into your autumn years. A life of wonder and beauty is possible to you if you choose that life which is the height of success—becoming the best person you have it in yourself to be.

The road to success and happiness is greatly simplified when we realize that within each of us already exists the seeds of a beautiful and rewarding life. These seeds await only the hand of nourishment and training before they burst out of their confining shell and blossom into maturity. This is true of us all. Shortly before George Bernard Shaw died, he was asked: "Mr. Shaw, you have known all the great men of your time—the artists, the writers, the statesmen. You have known royalty, you have wined and dined with those who have shaped the destiny of the world during your generation. Now, if you could be born again and relive your life as anyone of your choice, who would it be?"

Without a moment's hesitation, Shaw said, "If I could relive my life in the role of any person I desired, I would want to be the man George Bernard Shaw could have been, but was not."

Here is a man who by all ordinary standards of performance was among the greatest of his time. Yet he was dissatisfied. He realized how much more he could have done.

How satisfied are you with your life up to this point? If you could live it over again would you do it differently? We believe that most people, and we include ourselves in this number, would undoubtedly welcome outside help if they had it to do over. Although we cannot relive life's beginning, we can, beginning now, change its outcome. It is this belief which forms the rationale for this book.

In the chapters which follow we will present the beliefs and systems of conduct which we have learned from our experiences. Also, we will liberally call on Other People's Experience. Our guides will be selected not only from the great thinkers of our civilization but also from our own contemporaries. Their insights will illuminate your path.

A successful life can still be yours through decision and venture. Do not seek permission from others before setting out on the road to sui generis. You are responsible for your own life. You are responsible for your own choice. When you freely choose to get off the beaten path you will be rewarded by a freedom dimly glimpsed by the tardy or the timid. To squander your allotted span of life on this beautiful planet through doubt and indecision is too heavy a punishment. We are told in the Bible that, "Happy is the man that findeth wisdom, and the man that getteth understanding." Begin now to seek your own truth.

CHAPTER 2
THE TIME OF YOUR LIFE

"None are so old as those who have outlived their enthusiasm".
Thoreau

Throw away your stereotypes. The world of the next century will be radically different from the world of your past, and light years away from the world of your parents. It is human nature to bring the solutions of yesterday to the problems of today. Neither will be appropriate to the options of tomorrow. The rewards and the problems of the industrial age will not be transmitted into the next century. America is entering into the information age, and in this time of transition the qualities which will be needed for success are limited neither by sex nor by age: these qualities are knowledge, and people skills, and entrepreneurial ability, all of which are enhanced by age. So, miraculously, in your retirement years you will have an opportunity unprecedented in the history of civilization—at sixty years old you will have the same opportunity in the marketplace as a twenty-one year old, IF you are willing to make the same preparation. And you will have time to profit from it.

The world of the information age will differ from the world of the industrial age in ways so startling as to be indescribable. The world of the autumn of your life is apt to be to the world of your spring and summer as quantum mechanics is to Newtonian physics. Although the universe toward which we are headed cannot be pictured in terms of the stereotypes of our most recent decades, your own experience will be the reality which will guide you well in the years that lie ahead. As in quantum mechanics, the very act of observation changes the perceived reality. To make adequate preparation for this journey into new territory, it is instructive to get the broadest education possible concerning the world in which you will live. The years of your autumn afford the opportunity to look at the planet that is your whirling vehicle, and to look at it through eyes which are still open to the wonders of the world.

The information age to which the world is turning will bring with it a way of life in which the person over fifty can literally begin again with a high probability of success. This success can come from the fortuitous match of individual talent and temperament to the choice of endeavor. The industrial age, of which America was the leading nation, was biased in favor of physical strength, because it was physical strength which was required to run the mighty farms and factories that were the backbone of our nation. But the world has changed. The information age will depend on other qualities: the ability to reason, the ability to persuade others, the ability to communicate. Success will be knowledge-specific, and jobs will be highly specialized. The age that utilizes the laser beam and the opinion poll will accommodate an unimagined variety of vocations and of avocations. When you retire you will be in the luxurious position of structuring a future in which your success need not depend on physical power but on skill.

You can take the fear out of retirement through knowledge. You prepared for your current career through formal education; then you climbed the career ladder through the education born of experience. Successful retirement requires a comparable amount of education. This time the prize may be sweeter, for you will be preparing for work you *want* to do. But the requirements for education remain. You must prepare in triplicate—for physical health, financial health, and mental health. The learning that accompanies this preparation will not only remove your fears of the future, it will improve your life.

Neither health nor wealth is acquired overnight. To place your hopes for future happiness on the spinning wheel of chance is the equivalent of expecting to hold a winning ticket in an extravagantly unlikely lottery. The probability of pay-off approaches zero. Rather, health and wealth are acquired through knowledge translated into action, and action channelled into accomplishment.

Your avocation can become your vocation. You can measure your profit in this vocation in terms of financial gain, or people served, or simply your own knowledge of a job well done. If you choose to spend your time in the development of a talent which is already yours, and if you approach this use of your talent with the zest which comes from earned accomplishment, your retirement decades can be profitable beyond measure. You will truly be able to describe them as the best time of your life.

Your first career was as apt to have been decided by others as it was by you. How many of us chose our life's work by carefully and systematically matching our skills to our career choice? More likely, for most of us, choices were thrust upon us by the expectations of others. In many cases, we simply chose the jobs afforded by the geography of our home town. Lacking the imagination or the sense of adventure to strike out beyond the boundaries of our known environment, most of us settled for a reassuring sameness in our lives. If the assurance settled slowly into the ruts of routine, most of us were too busy to notice the precise moment of the shift. Many of us literally gave our lives to the company store.

But retirement compels change. When change is mandatory, does it not seem desirable that we should all want to structure the change toward happiness? You will no longer be required to work for your daily bread. The retirement benefits earned through long years of your first career will assure that you are able to put bread on your retirement table. Your choice of the use you make of the freedom of your future will decide whether you will be able to buy butter for your bread and hyacinths for your soul.

The structure of your future can be built through the technique of situational analysis. Using this technique you can answer the questions:
1. Who am I?
2. What do I want to do?
3. Why do I want to do it?
4. How am I going to do it?

In this book we will help you design your own strategic plan to answer your questions. In effect, we will help you analyze how you can effect change to assure a good future. When you look at your own future from a marketing perspective, you will make your future plans based on your known strengths and opportunities. You will list your strengths and realistically acknowledge your liabilities. You will define any obstacles to your plans, and assess your major opportunities. The essence of problem solving consists of understanding all the elements of the situation, and in clearly defining the problem. The first question to be asked is, "Am I doing the right thing?" The second is, "Am I doing the right thing right?" We shall address these questions in detail in later chapters.

In framing your future, it is time to concentrate on your identity, coming to terms with who you are, what you can do, what you hope to do in the future. You need not only to understand yourself, but also to understand your relationship to the community of which you are a part. Your identity can be defined in two different sets: strengths which are internal, and those which are dependent on the external and larger world. Internal strengths are composed of experience, education, wisdom, character, our concept of unique personhood. External strengths include the professional or business networks of your career, your public service associations, the reputation of the firms for which you have worked, your family, and circle of friends. Past successes in both these sets will clarify your sense of your strengths and form a basis for your future accomplishments.

Identity experts tell us that people who are facing retirement are especially vulnerable. People who have gotten their sense of identity primarily from their jobs are likely to have external identities, which are representative of their status to the world. People who have measured their lives in percentage of sales, or patients served, or portfolios built, may define themselves primarily by their work. But these external measures tell little about the person inside, and will vanish at retirement. Often, before retirement, these people begin to feel a sense of isolation and aloneness. If your work has been your identity, you must now come to terms with your personal strengths. The identity that is critical to your freedom years is internal.

In all of your planning you will be conscious of the passing of time. Because the moments are so precious in the golden years, it is of the utmost importance that you learn how to capture the moment, the "fragment of eternity."

Perhaps the most famous riddle in all mythology is that posed in one of Voltaire's writings:

"What is the longest and yet the shortest?
The swiftest and yet the slowest.
All of us neglect it. Then we all regret it.
Nothing can be done without it.
It swallows up all that is small
And it builds up all that is great?"

The answer, of course, is time.

Time is the longest because it is the measure of eternity. It is the shortest because none of us has time to finish life's work. It is swift to those who are happy, slow to those who suffer. We all neglect it and consequently regret it. Nothing can be done without it, for it is the only theatre in which we live.

It swallows up into oblivion all that is unworthy of posterity, and it builds and preserves for immortality all that is great and unselfish.

One of the oldest techniques for success is this: A successful man spends his time forming the habit of doing things that the failure is unwilling to do. Psychologists tell us this is because the average man finds it easier to adjust to the hardships of the familiar than to spend the time adjusting to the sacrifices that lead to success in the untried. For too many, known evils are preferable to the risks associated with the unknown.

Each day we have the opportunity to deal with the miracle of time—time, life's most valuable commodity. Time is that priceless gift whose value cannot be weighed in the balance or tested in the crucible. No plumb line can sound its depth of importance; no ladder can scale its heights. Time is the sole ingredient through which we can transform our dreams into reality—our visions into success. Killing time is not a simple crime—it is murder. Time is so precious that the creator in his infinite wisdom gives it to us in small doses so that we cannot squander it. We cannot store it up; we can only use it as it is given to us; and we can only use the present. The past is truly only prologue—the future is yet to be.

Yesterday is a cancelled check; tomorrow is a promissory note; only today is legal tender—only *now* is negotiable. The best effect of this or any other book is that it motivates the reader to take action. If our words can motivate you to take the action of learning to live every day, they will have served their purpose. In Shakespeare's words:

"For yesterday is but a dream and tomorrow is
  only a vision,
But today well lived makes every yesterday a
  dream of happiness
And every tomorrow a vision of hope.
Look well, therefore, to this day
Such is the salutation to the dawn."

Each day we all start out with the same amount of time. Our daily purses are magically filled with twenty-four hours of that infinitely precious substance we call life. Nature is no respecter of persons. The hands of the clock turn around at the same speed for each of us. For some, the meaning of time is that when opportunity is at its highest. The word "opportunity" itself, was inspired by the idea of proper timing. It is derived from the Latin *ab portu*, meaning literally, "out of port." In the centuries before modern ports, ships would congregate off the shore waiting for high tide before bringing their goods to shore in smaller boats. The crews that took alert advantage of the time and arrived at the market place first were able to obtain the best prices for their cargo. Those which were lazy, complacent, or late in bringing their cargo to market were the losers. This formed the background for Shakespeare's writing:

"There is a tide in the affairs of men
Which, taken at the flood, leads on to Fortune;
Omitted, all the voyage of their life
Is bound in shallows and in miseries."

The time when opportunity is most favorable has special significance to many. In bullfighting it is called the moment of truth; in sales it is the instant the salesman receives the "closing signal." Advertising people tell us that there is nothing as powerful as an idea whose time has arrived—a need that has finally become apparent. If you can learn to recognize the right moment when it comes, the problems of life become vastly simplified. The Old Testament tells us of the timeliness of happenings, "To everything there is a season, and a time to every matter under heaven." In this season of your life it is time to follow the valedictory of your retirement with your personal salutation to the dawn!

If you decide to make the autumn of your life your most successful years you will learn to appreciate time's most important dimensions, its depth. The horizontal dimension of time is the shallowest of concepts. No great masterpieces were created, no great music composed, no great discoveries produced by those who gave importance to this concept. This perception of time is tragic because it destroys initiative and discourages creative impulses. Actually, we all have a great amount of time—nature has generously endowed us. It is simply a matter of what we consider important enough to do during the hours which belong to us. The people who give real meaning to life and make the world a better place are those who give the great quality of depth to time. It is the dimension of depth which gives real substance to life.

When Cavett is speaking from the platform he has the time of his life. With fire in his eyes and intensity in his soul, he is doing what he loves to do—teaching, preaching, and persuading. Last year, at age 78, he made 150 speeches. He enjoyed audiences from Alaska to Australia, Hong Kong, Singapore, and New Zealand, in addition to criss-crossing the cities of America. His message has consistently been, "We're in the People Business," and Cavett practices what he preaches. When he is joined with his audience in that magnetic meshing of minds which is at the heart of platform speaking, he is a happy man. He feels that he has tapped the source of the fountain of youth. In these moments he agrees with Browning that this is the best, the last for which the first was made.

Fortunate are the persons for whom time is no longer imprisoned by the clock or shackled by the calendar. Their lives are governed by dedication and enthusiasm—not by days or hours or weeks. Their convictions have come alive, and their days are filled with zest. They believe so strongly in what they are doing that they are drawn toward their goals by a powerful magnetic force which does not even recognize time. Paradoxically, these are the people for whom time appears to stand still. Their appearance is youthful, their voice is hopeful, and their outlook is cheerful. When the heart is harnessed to a task that is loved, work is a mission. This is your challenge; to defy time by refusing to be imprisoned by its limitations.

The Kansas City Star featured a story about a man who is living a life that would make many people turn green with envy. As the editor stated in his summary column:

"Who is this Speedy, the subject of this week's column cover story? And what kind of lesson does he teach? He parties every night. He hangs around with fellow musicians until all hours. He sashays about with people one-third his age. He plays drums. He sings. All of this at the age of 73...Speedy has chosen a different path. To become a drummer to a different march, as it were. At 73, Speedy has chosen to become the platonic escort for a consort of women who might pass for University of California cheerleaders. Speedy has chosen to jam in murky nightclubs, to tell ribald stories to his friends, to start his own band, and to chat amiably with nightcritters and music lovers in ten counties until the sun comes up. In short, Speedy has chosen, here in the boiling uncertainties of 20th century life, to dally. The result is that he sleeps well, smiles, sings, plays, and finally, judges not his fellow man."

And from his story a picture of a happy man emerges. In the hours after midnight, when jams form the backdrop for men seeking courage and women ready for friendship, Speedy is in his element. Nearly all the regulars in town know him, those eternal optimists who chase the good life. Most have affectionate stories about him. When he walks into the clubs the men shake his hand, the women hug him or lay an affectionately familiar hand on his arm to remind him of other times. More often than not he is asked to sit in with band or to croon a favorite request. He is the consummate old pro. From the late 1920's through the forties and fifties he sang, danced, played the drums and lived it up in big dance halls across the country.

There followed years of more conventional employment, working for the Office of Disease Control, and after that the Veterans Administration. Even now, at age 73, Speedy is a part-time social worker. He helps the elderly and disabled and he finds the work rewarding. But his real life begins much later in the day.

Six months ago he became a bandleader for the first time. He was asked to play a regular gig at one of Kansas City's well known jazz clubs. He plays drums and sings, holding a mike in one hand and stirring the brushes with the other. His touch with the brushes and his touch with a tune are equally sure, and the sound is vintage jazz. The youngest man in his combo is 69. Like Speedy, their technique is terrific. Nobody can swing like the old cats.

In one of Ann Landers' columns, she pointed out that many artists, musicians, scientists, and writers did their best work when they were in their 60s, 70s or 80s. Goethe completed Faust after he was 80. Amos Alonzo Stagg was still coaching football when he was 100. The list includes Grandma Moses, Winston Churchill, Vladimir Horowitz, Pablo Picasso, Frank Lloyd Wright, Georgia O'Keefe, Carl

Sandburg, George Burns, Bob Hope, Grace Hopper, and Albert Einstein. Will you add your name to this list?

CHAPTER 3
BEYOND MATERIALISM

"For what doth it profit a man if he gain the whole world, and lose his own soul?" Holy Bible

There are a lot of us now of retirement age who were adroitly led down the primrose path during the decades of the 1950s-1970s. Astutely guided by our major industries, we began to believe that the good life could be bought in the marketplace. Our social codes and our personal goals were too often shaped by the mass media. And, for many, our youthfully romantic dreams were offered up in willing substitutions for materialistic maturity.

The lovely young girls who at 18 were immersed in dreams of moonlight and roses were transformed within a decade into competitive production managers. Dutiful housewives, they engaged in spirited neighborhood competition over whose wash had the whitest bleach, whose floor the brightest shine, whose children the most advantages. Their husbands matched their competitiveness. While their wives began to design an attempt at family living modeled on the living color of television, the men gave themselves to their careers. Youthful idealism was replaced by conditions more substantial: comfort, competence, and—for many—a search for certainty through possessions.

In an atomic age, our generation began our search for certainty in a precariously uncertain world. Lacking a global perspective, and beguiled by the demands of our families and careers, we paid insufficient attention to the many problems and needs of our country. Moving our home and families according to the demands of an expanding economy, we based many of our judgments upon external evidence. The country expanded in prosperity, and the goals of our maturity were based on possessions.

We sought and found the good life. For many, the price we paid was the sublimation of our youthful dreams. We substituted corporate goals for our own. But we did not find certainty, and we did not find security.

We launched a consumer economy in America. We enjoyed the highest standard of living, the most expansive careers, the largest number of children yet recorded in this country. We may be the last generation that sublimated individual dreams to the greater good of corporation and family. We have been rewarded by an unprecedented Gross National Product, and we have earned the right to resume the dreams of our youth. In our freedom years, life can be measured in finer stuff than our possessions.

During the decades when we were occupied with our lives, America lost her place as the world's greatest industrial nation. Identity consultant Beverly Bubeck analyzes our situation as follows: "During the Vietnam War, America lost her identity because she lost sight of what was important. There is a direct relationship between the identity of us as individuals and that of us as a nation because the health of any society is dependent on the health of individuals."

Our generation has had the best of America. We have the opportunity now to pay for our privileges with the coin of responsibility. Children of the depression, we were formed by the desperate Thirties, the war-torn Forties, and the decades of prosperity that followed. We have been both dutiful and responsible. Even now, in retirement, our responsibilities remain a part of the pattern of our lives. For some, responsibilities and pride of place may define our next few decades. Many in retirement will turn to work on the problems of this country as a way of repaying a personal debt to the blessings of democracy.

On all sides there is work to be done. Our public education system needs massive overhaul. Our municipal and state governments are expensive and inefficient. Crime threatens us all. We need far better child care. Our generation, free now from the necessity to spend most of our waking hours in making a living, can choose to work to change the downward drift of our magnificent country.

Few of us will deny its magnificence. We retain from the air we breathed in our childhood a zealous pride of place and spirit that transcends our current woes and worries concerning America. We have for too long taken for granted this sense of pride and affection for America's geographic and spiritual environment. Taken for granted, also, are the warmth, the decency, and the energy which are the typical characteristics of our upbringing. To say that we are patriotic because our country has been good to us is at once too simplistic and too self-serving a reason. Our love of country goes far beyond these surface attributes. The essence of our deep feeling for America must be found in an analysis of what really counts. Principles count. Hard work counts. Optimism counts. Freedom counts. Our old confidence that we were citizens of the greatest industrial nation in the world has been replaced by a pragmatic view that we must examine our past premises in order to shore up our future. It is here that we of retirement age can exert our efforts to help build a future which will be a worthy legacy for our descendants.

Perhaps we can prepare for service to others and to our own country through study, getting in touch with the patriotism and love of country which form the ground of altruistic public service. Few deny that the need for unselfish public service exists in our time. While America and Americans have taken for granted the many blessings which made the good life possible for those of our generation, we are now in grave danger of allowing erosion of the basic structure of our civilization. Whether this erosion is allowed to continue will depend in great measure on the assumption of responsibility of the only leisure class left in America—those who have reached the age of retirement. The authors believe that there is no better way to justify our existence on this beautiful planet than to resolve in the autumn of our lives to assume the responsibility of citizenship. Patriotism and love of country alone are insufficient. Just as faith without works is ineffective, a professed belief in democracy needs informed action to insure its success. Will you resolve in your retirement years to change and improve those structures basic to a democracy—education, government?

Ours may be the last generation which encloses in our collective memory the self-sufficient attitude bred on the American frontier. The legacy handed down to us from our forefathers is a proud one, a legacy where privilege and talent were repaid through public service. To be idle in our retirement would be to squander the infinite riches available to us through service to the larger community. As we examine the lists of woes which now exist we can find ample use for all our talents. To direct our intelligence, our energy, our accumulated wisdom toward a solution of even one of America's major problems would constitute a magnificent memorial. Our talents are diverse. There is strength in diversity when it is channeled wisely. It is our hope that the wisdom and talents which are the endowment of America's retirees will be translated into a renaissance in this country.

If we do this, we must take advantage of our opportunity to assess the design of our own lives in terms of the quality of our dreams. We now can ask the fundamental question, "Is my life worthy of my dreams?"

While our dreams may have shifted over the years, retirement brings with it the maturity and the opportunity to structure a civilization in support of our dreams. The materialism of our middle years has made possible that rarest of privileges—the privilege of cultivating the larger human values.

No longer need we measure our accomplishments against unrelenting standards of prosperity, parenthood, social life and sexuality clearly beyond the capabilities of most of us. As we move in retirement toward suigeneris, we can let go of the search for certainty through consumerism. Rather, we can examine more thoroughly the stuff of which a truly good life is made. If we can do this, then we can help America take a significant step forward. It is not too much to hope that each of us can move beyond materialism toward courage and compassion and common sense—and even toward love, that truest of profits.

CHAPTER 4
WHAT DOES YOUR FUTURE HOLD?

"Nature seems to exist for the excellent." Ralph Waldo Emerson.

Your future offers you the freedom to become your real self. There are five requirements for the best of all futures:
1. You must learn to love the world around you.
2. You must learn what makes you happy.
3. You must learn where your true strengths and talents lie.
4. You must learn to make decisions that are true to yourself.
5. You must work to carry out these decisions.

We are formed by the geography of our past, separated like continents by our own experiences. The winds of fate which have changed our own lives have altered the lives of those around us to various degrees, some small, some enormous. It is idle to say that we are alike. We are different people, each with singular genetic inheritances, talents, and temperaments. We share qualities of the mind and the body, yet we remain separate and unique, a tribute to the infinite variety imaginable only to the creator. So it follows that when we optimize our talents, physical, mental, and spiritual, we will have attained the quality of suigeneris—becoming our unique and best selves.

We are the product of the questions we have asked in the past. Our future depends on the questions we ask ourselves now. These are simple questions. It is the answers that are difficult, for our lives are framed by our responses. Certainly, these are key questions that should be asked:
1. What are your major talents?
2. What does it take to make you happy?
3. What is your ultimate goal?

We shall consider these questions separately.

Question One: What are your major talents?

We are all full of possibilities, but this we know to be true: We cannot accomplish anything greater than that which we are.

The picture is no greater than the artist, the book no greater than its writer, the music no greater than the composer. Human laws are as certain as the laws of nature, and nature deals with severe impartiality. Water cannot rise above its source; the seedlings of oak trees do not produce weeds.

The results we obtain can be no greater than the qualities and talents which are contained within us. Ralph Waldo Emerson defined this law precisely when he wrote, "Use what language you will, you can never say anything but what you are."

Once we have accepted this great human law, we have simplified our search for excellence and clarified the choices which will define our future. People who are inspired by ambition but restrained by indolence struggle futilely to improve their circumstances rather than improve themselves. Too many of us have spent our lives looking for a better JOB, or hoping for a fortunate chance, without disciplining ourselves in order to DO A BETTER JOB with the talents which lie ready to our hands.

It is one of the profound truths of life that we ought constantly to engage in self analysis with honesty and humility. And as we grow in self understanding we ought to discipline ourselves toward the fullest use of the powers and talents that we discover within us. The joy that comes from the full use of our own talents is more precious than rubies, and even more rare.

Since the beginning of time there have been two groups of people. The first, and by far the larger group, is composed of the many who look for a way of life which is not too demanding, one that makes little claim on their capabilities. These are the ones who will sit out their retirement years dying on the installment plan. But the major work of the world is done by those in the smaller group, those ambitious and resourceful people who continuously seek to prepare themselves for the greater tasks and opportunities of life. Those who seek the easier way have always failed, the ease of mediocrity accelerating their slide to the bottom. Only those who seek strength to meet the challenges of life become our leaders. Robert Frost said that the world is full of willing people; some willing to work, the rest willing to let them.

Only the difficult offers a real challenge, for the great task of life is to use all of our talents to their true potential. Phillips Brooks crystallized this principle in language of precision: "Do not pray for tasks equal to your powers. Pray for powers equal to your tasks. Then the doing of your work shall be no miracle, but you shall be the miracle."

Just as we cannot repeal the law of gravity, neither can we repeal this law of man's behavior: we cannot accomplish anything except that which we are. It follows that if we aspire to excellence we need to become the best person we have it in us to be.

The work is improved by improving the workman. The painting is improved by inspiring the artist. And the sermon cannot be any greater than the character of the speaker. What you are does, indeed, speak more loudly than what you say.

Question Two: What does it take to make you happy?

Unhappy people wish their lives away, convinced that if only they could move from point A where they are now, to point B, some point fixed on the path ahead, their happiness would come automatically as soon as they reached point B. Happy people know to seek happiness from the journey, going beyond point B to other vistas.

There is great freedom to be found in the future. Each of us has a past framed by a unique combination of forces. Our future will be built by another set of forces and decisions. We can choose to build on the skills which are ours, those talents and experiences which will combine to bring out the best that is in us. The inevitable end of life is beyond our power to determine, but the journey of life itself can be fresh and hopeful and fruitful.

The secret lies in deciding to be happy. The arts of seers and fortune tellers notwithstanding, our futures are not already molded, waiting for us to discover them, like plastic marvels pre-fabricated in a cosmic amusement park. Rather, our futures are before us in infinite variety, and the permutations of our choices are breathtaking. The happiest people are those who refuse to become bitter about those matters over which they have no control, those matters which lie in their past. Absorbing all their experiences as a part of the immensely rich fabric of life, happy people transcend their obstacles and grow and gain strength through the journey.

One of the happiest men we met during our interviews was a man who had learned this lesson the hard way. Now the director of the music program for a community college, Sam, in his early sixties, considers himself to be a fortunate man. The day we met him, Sam was auditioning students for the newly formed jazz ensemble, absorbed in the rhythms and improvisations of the musicians who would be his students. Later that same day he would meet with the community chorus for the first time that semester. His head was filled with music and his face was alive with excitement.

Until three years ago, Sam was one of the leading swine producers in the nation. He had owned and operated a hog farm so outstanding that it had been featured in farm magazines as a national model. He and his family had lived the good life, with every expectation of passing on to his sons the farm Sam had inherited and expanded. But he had not reckoned with the national farm crisis set in motion by the economic policies of the early 1980's. Facing economic ruin when he was sixty, he found himself sliding from affluence to bankruptcy, irresistibly propelled by world-wide economic forces. His personal skill as a farmer and community leader proved insufficient to ward off economic disaster.

Sustained by the love of his family and the respect of all who knew him, Sam began the process of structuring the rest of his life. The first question he asked himself was, "What does it take to make me happy?" He reviewed his life from childhood, through college, through his years of maturity, and realized that a continuous thread of joy had been provided by music. He had been an award-winning drummer in high school, had played in the marching band through college, had sung in choirs since early childhood, and had directed the choir at his country church for the past thirty years.

Translating this analysis into action, he earned a second degree in two years at the state university, secured a part-time teaching position at his local community college, and entered his freedom third. For Sam, the road beyond affluence was the road to suigeneris.

Resolve that in this next third of your life you, too, will be happy. Abraham Lincoln was absolutely right when he said, "Most people are about as happy as they make up their minds to be." Discipline yourself not to dwell on the thoughts that lead to depression. Consciously remove them from your mind and replace them with constructive thoughts. Retirement offers you the opportunity to improve your mind by studying the things which are truly of interest to you. Learn the techniques of replacing unhappy thoughts with study or with constructive action. Face your fears, and gather the courage to go past them. As true today as it ever was when Pericles spoke to the Athenians, the secret of happiness is, indeed, a brave heart. Become acquainted with your own heart.

Your freedom years will not be free, and you will not be happy, until you listen to your inner voice. This voice is framed by your own unique consciousness, the voice that speaks only to you. Have you listened to it lately? Or has it been muffled by custom and duty, grown rusty through neglect and disuse? The heart has its reasons, and is entitled to be heard.

Question Three: What is your ultimate goal?

It was Bertrand Russell who wrote that three passions had governed his life: the longing for love, the search for knowledge, and pity for the sufferings of mankind. These passions defined his goals. And your passions will define yours. Whether you aspire to the nobility of purpose of a saint or a scientist, or whether you ask simply to tend your own garden in peaceful solitude, your success in retirement will be measured by the relationship between your life and your goals. Whether you measure your success in terms of knowledge acquired, or services rendered, or people loved, or wealth attained, it is you who will ultimately determine whether your life has been a success. Your retirement will be a success if you live your life so as to use to full measure that which is contained within you. To set your goals in the pursuit of excellence using the talents which are already yours, is to set your sights on becoming the best you have it in you to be.

Picture in your mind the person you could become if you used to the fullest all those talents which are already yours. Picture the person you could be if you became yourself. The search for a rewarding future begins with you. When you accept the responsibility of becoming the person you already have it in you to be, you will have taken the first step on the most rewarding journey of your life. Design your own best path, acknowledge your own strengths, and choose the happiness that is earned through effort. The traits which are already a part of your heritage form the foundation for the future which can be yours.

You are creating your future now. You can make it what you choose.

II. METHODS

CHAPTER 5
DECIDE WHAT YOU REALLY WANT

"Enjoy to the full the resources that are within thy reach."
Pindar

The method described in this chapter is meant to help you design a new career path in which you will have fun while making a profit. Work without enjoyment is dreary: enjoyment without profit may be a luxury you cannot afford. The techniques listed here will acquaint you with your selves—the self you were as a child, the self you were as a teenager and young adult, and the self you have become in maturity. You will receive clues about your inner self as you review the patterns of your life.

First, Seek the Pattern:
1. Check your Happiness Chart:
   Begin by keeping a record of your emotional temperature. Each day for the next 90 days take the time at the end of the day to fill out this simple form.
   Review your day in your mind, and check your remembered emotions. How did you feel in the morning? Were you happy, or not happy, or somewhere in between? Put a check mark under the emotion that best describes your morning mood. Then do the

same for your afternoon and evening. Do this quickly, without interpretation. This should not take more than two minutes per day, including the time it takes to record any comment you wish to write at the bottom of the form. Please take the time to make yourself a set of cards. Ordinary three by five cards will do fine. So will pieces of paper with the same form copied on each. This is your chart to record your happiness quotient:

TABLE I: Your Happiness Chart

DATE	HAPPY	SO-SO	NOT HAPPY	WHERE WERE YOU?	WHO WAS WITH YOU?	WHAT WERE YOU DOING?
Morning						
Afternoon						
Evening						

WRITE ANY COMMENTS ABOUT THE DAY:

At the end of ninety days gather all ninety cards and study them to find the pattern of your emotions. Begin by sorting out all the cards that were checked happy. Spread these out as you would a big deck of cards and study the patterns of your happiness. What were you doing that made you happy? Who was with you? Can you see a pattern? Some of you will find that you are made happy by the occupations afforded by geography, skiing in the mountains, or fishing in gulf stream waters. Others will be reminded of what they already knew, that the company of special people will make the difference between happiness and apathy. But for most, happiness is more complex, and, fortunately, more available. Most people will list many activities, places for happiness, and will see the possibilities of permutations of these.

Now, look at your cards again, this time sorting out those cards which were marked unhappy. Analyze these the same way, paying attention to those factors which keep recurring on your unhappiness cards. If you are one of those unfortunate individuals whose cards were seldom checked for happiness, consider the probability that you have been spending your time in the wrong way, in the wrong place, with the wrong people!

Ponder the pattern which has emerged, and begin to consider how you can choose another career, one that will allow you to do what you already enjoy doing; one that you know something about, and one that will allow you to make some money in the process.

2. Reacquaint Yourself with Your Selves:

A. Take an ordinary notebook and write in it the answers to these questions:

> Describe yourself as a child:

1. What did you look like?
2. Where did you live?
3. What did you enjoy?
4. Whom did you love?
5. What did you daydream about?
6. Who were your friends?
7. What did you want to do when you grew up?

Take a few minutes to picture in your mind the child you were then. Reach back in your memory and try to imagine that child, the one who is still within.

B. *Describe yourself as a teenager and young adult:*

1. What did you look like?
2. When were you happy?
3. What did you worry about?

4. How did you spend your spare time?
   5. How did you earn your spending money?
   6. What did you daydream about?
   7. What did you expect out of life?
   8. Whom did you envy?
   9. Whom did you pattern yourself after?
  10. Who influenced you the most?

Take a few minutes to recapture the feelings of that young person. How many of your expectations have you realized? How much of that youthful zest can you still feel today when you are happy? How much of it would you like to recapture?

   C. *Now describe your present self*:
   1. What do you look like?
   2. Whom do you love?
   3. Where do you live?
   4. According to the marks on your happiness temperature chart, what do you enjoy doing the most?
   5. What do you dislike the most?
   6. What do you daydream about?
   7. What do you want out of life?

Study the answers to this last set of questions, and compare them with those of your childhood and youth. Have you shifted your sights? Has this shift been a good one? Do you begin to see some patterns in common among these seasons of your life?

3. Now is the time for analysis of your strengths and talents. Please answer the questions which follow in as objective a fashion as possible.

What are the strengths that describe your character and personality? What are your competencies? Please make four lists:

TABLE II: Your List of Strengths

1. *Things I do Very Well*

2. *Things I do Moderately Well*

3. *Character Strengths*

4. *Personality Strengths*

What would you like to do better?

4. The remainder of the questions will help you focus on your present life while providing clues as to how you can design your future.
    How important is love to you?
    How important is respect to you?
    How important is recognition to you?
    How important is money to you?
    How many obligations do you have to others?
    What do you like most about your present life?
    What do you dislike most about it?
    What do you do for pleasure?
    How often are you bored?
    Which of your skills give you the most pleasure?

Take the time now to catch a glimpse of the future which could be yours if you could design a business or profession which would use those skills which give you pleasure. Let the idea of using these skills in service to others take root in your mind. Begin now the study of specialized situations which will usefully and profitably fit into the world of tomorrow.

Let your mind accept the idea of success in these new ventures. Begin now to spend time each day in the study of the profitable interactions of your talents with the needs of others in the future which will be the information age.

It was Cavett's post-retirement review of his own talents which gave rise to the National Speakers Association. Retiring from the practice of law at the age of sixty-one, Cavett found that he had shut the door on his career and opened the door to boredom. As he recalls it, after six weeks of retirement he felt himself to be dying on the installment plan, a victim of infectious apathy. Concluding that he would have to act as his own physician, he set about designing a cure. The habits of analysis and synthesis ingrained by decades of legal work were his tools in his diagnosis. The symptoms were simple, but the cure was complex.

Cavett began his search by reviewing his past, looking for the threads of joy which had enriched his life. Even as a schoolboy he had loved public speaking. The youngest child in a competitive family defined by academic tradition, he had been expected to enter a profession and to excel in it. This expectation had been a part of his choice of the profession of law. The love for oratory which he shared with his brothers was a part of his heritage. Challenge and change were his preferred environment.

Propelled from Starkville, Mississippi, to a glamourous Wall Street law firm via Washington and Lee University, Cavett exuberantly adapted to the excitement of New York City. When he was loaned by his firm to the District Attorney's office to work on Tom Dewey's racket investigation team, he was in his element. As was always to be the case, he thrived on analysis, action, and the excitement of being in the people business.

When health problems mandated a move to Phoenix, Arizona, Cavett found the elements of success waiting his catalytic hand. In 1937, Phoenix had 42,000 people. It was ready for the enthusiastic leadership of a civic-minded attorney. Always more interested in his clients' sales problems than in their legal problems, Cavett played the role of community organizer. He helped build the National Tennis Patron Association, the Sombrero Theatre, the Boy's Club, the Blood Bank, the Heart Association. He built three country clubs, and become so involved in the development of surrounding real estate that some said he could have slowed the growth of Phoenix by refusing to sell any more of it. The years of frenetic activity formed the pattern of his life. Small wonder that retirement brought a crash landing to a high-flying career. In retrospect, Cavett is amazed that he did not foresee the inevitable boredom in a retirement which was supposed to be devoted to the leisure he had not previously enjoyed.

His retirement had not been based on his customary analysis. Rather, he had scheduled retirement in conformance with the unexamined assumptions which governed the lives of his peers. For the first 61 years of his life, Cavett lived according to the rules of the world around him, rules which he had assumed were both useful and mandatory. But at 61 he decided that life could be determined by selectivity. Real happiness, he believes, is found by bursting out of the shell designed for the many. Real happiness is an individual matter. For Cavett, happiness came from selecting the things to do that he enjoyed the most, then giving himself the freedom to do them. At retirement he gave himself the joy of using full time those talents to which he had formerly given a small portion of his time.

After Cavett had studied how he wanted to blend his own talents, he concluded that he really enjoyed promotion, motivation, speaking, and teaching. This blend produced the Phoenix Summer Sales Seminars, a small school designed to teach people how to speak and how to sell. At that time there was a heavy distrust of the profession of public speaking, with most firms preferring to conduct their own training sessions rather than use outside speakers. Cavett set out to change this preference. The first year Cavett enrolled 16 students, the second year 60, and the third year, 200. From that time forward, it became a matter of managing the growth of the new enterprise, which in 1973 was incorporated as the National Speakers Association. The Association now has more than 2,500 members. Cavett has blended his organizational ability, his speaking skills, and his flair for salesmanship to found a new profession.

Cavett's advice is a simple prescription: take inventory, select the things you enjoy, and blend them to suit yourself. There is no one on this earth who is better equipped to determine your aims in life than you, yourself. You are your own authority, and you have earned this right through long decades of coming to terms with yourself and the world about you. The great tragedy of life is that too many people go through life and never sing the song they are born to sing. The game of life is ready to be played when you are ready. Think of retirement not as your leave taking but as your beginning—the beginning of that part of your life in which you will become your true self. Plan to play the game of life. Just as the postscript is the most important part of a letter, so can the post retirement years become the most important part of your life. Make your freedom years memorable by blending your talents in the pursuit of happiness.

One of the greatest changes in the last 40 years in our whole economic system has occurred in the field of retirement. As is so often the case, our philosophies have not kept pace with current reality. At a time when American adults enjoy unprecedented health and life expectancies, we cling to the outworn assumptions appropriate to generations past.

The man who retired at the turn of the century had a life expectancy of two years. His plans quite appropriately included rest and leisure. The man or woman of today who anticipates 20 years of good health would do well to design a new beginning. Twenty years is too long to sit on any shelf, no matter how comfortable.

We recently interviewed a beautiful woman who refuses to sit on the shelf at all.

Her posture would do credit to a duchess. Her figure is still a slim and trim size 10. Viewed from the back, only her silvery chignon betrays that she is a day over 40. When she turns and you see the faint lines in her lovely face you begin to make a more accurate guess as to her real age. Even so, you would miss it by a decade.

Ann's philosophy of life shows in her face, a patrician face which reflects a serene worldliness. You sense that she can ignore the second rate, rise above the petty, and discipline herself toward her own best interests. Her occupation is cause for astonishment. She operates the check room in a luxury hotel. At age 77, she is the hatcheck girl.

For more than twenty five years, Ann was an accomplished saleswoman of ladies clothing, working in a large city for a locally-owned specialty store of impressive reputation. When it closed Ann joined another fine store. By the time the second store had fought and lost the battle with chain department stores, she was eligible for social security checks. But she was unwilling to live the narrow life mandated by their restrictions.

A life of uninterrupted leisure is not to Ann's liking, anyway. It goes against her responsible upbringing. As she puts it, she hates the "What am I going to do today?" lifestyle. Living for luncheons and trips and television seems to her to be the shallowest of ways to spend time. She likes to interact with people and to have fun with people. One of the many skills she honed in her years as a saleswoman was that of successfully handling many different kinds of people. Sales work in a fine clothing store provides variety, the experience of dealing with a different customer every hour. Selling under these circumstances becomes a game of skill, a game at which Ann excelled.

She sees no merit in retiring to rest. Rest is near the bottom of her scale of values; she prefers the energizing effects of her three mile evening walk. Even now, she has no specific plans for retirement. Her work at the hotel adds flavor to her days. She likes the money, she likes her customers, and she has a good relationship with the management.

Ann's advice to persons designing a new lifestyle in retirement is sound. She suggests that most people would do better to change to a different but related field: "We get too stale if we stay put, too unwilling to learn new ways. Yet we should not make a change so radical that we don't understand the requirements of the new career. An experienced feel for what you are doing is the asset that can be transferred from one line of work to another."

Beautifully dressed, meticulously groomed, and totally poised, Ann concluded the interview and returned to her work.

We need a change in the whole philosophy of retirement. All of us start out excited over life's great venture. As young men and women we are eager to live life to the fullest; our dreams are vivid and our hopes are high. But most find out all too soon that somewhere between the reality in which we live and the great city of our dreams is a little town called compromise. Too many decide to make it their permanent home. These cities are not on any map. They are not listed in any census report, but they are just as much a part of your life as the city in which you live, pay taxes, and vote. How near your town of compromise is to your city of dreams depends on you. The preparation you make for your retirement years will determine whether you spend your time in your dream city or in the compromise town. If you begin realistically to lay your plans to move, your day of retirement can be your day of graduation.

All of life should be a required course in studying the joys of living. All of life is a preparation for release—not a release into the void of apathy, but the release into the full use of our talents.

The oak sleeps in the acorn,
The butterfly emerges from the cocoon,
And freedom is the dividend earned from duty.

CHAPTER 6
MATCH YOUR TALENTS TO YOUR TASK

"Hands are the heart's landscape." Pope John Paul II

Somewhere between living to work and working to live is a golden mean—working for fun *and* profit. As you set about the business of deciding what you want to do with the rest of your life, you need to come to terms with your feelings about work. What kinds of work have you enjoyed so far? At which of your career points have you been the happiest? What aspects of your most recent position have been the most fulfilling? What part of your job descriptions have you liked the least, or, worse yet, actively disliked?

The next set of exercises is designed to help you sort out your talents and to weave these into the pattern of your next career. At this stage of your life you need to pay a lot of attention to your talents, not only those which are yours through biological inheritance, but also those which have been developed through your interaction with the world around you. Look carefully at the traits you have displayed up until now to discover their common patterns through each of your jobs so far. It is not the duplication of these traits that we are seeking, but rather an analysis of their patterns. Our aim is to pay attention to the tendencies which are in your bones, and to emphasize those that bring you pleasure.

Our preferences and abilities can be separated into three broad categories: preference for working with ideas, preference for working with things, and preference for working with people. Most of us have strong abilities in one or two of these categories, and are rather weak in the third. Certainly we all have stronger preferences for one category than another. The shy person will often prefer to deal with ideas and with things—mechanical, technological, or artistic—rather than interacting with people. The extrovert with a strong mechanical aptitude may have little interest in the theoretical explanation of ideas.

Most of us have an instinctive knowledge of our own strengths. In the hope that her own mistakes will be somewhat instructive to others, Louise likes to tell the story of the mismatch between her own talents and her position requirements on her first job. Louise, an extrovert who gets caught up in the possibilities of ideas, admits to having less mechanical ability than anyone she has ever met. Her talent table looks like this:

LOUISE'S TALENT TABLE

Preferences for Working With:	High	Moderate	Low
People	x		
Ideas	x		
Things			x

When she graduated from college with a degree in mathematics, Louise was offered two jobs. The first was a teaching position which paid very little money. The other was a position as a computer (in those long ago days persons with calculators laboriously performed the mathematical computations now programmed into computers). This second position was in the seismographic office of a major oil company and paid exactly twice as much as the first. Louise promptly accepted the larger salary, and thus committed her days to the routine computation of velocity depth charts and their accompanying logarithmic and trigonometric calculations. For a lively and gregarious nineteen year old, the solitary confinement of her quiet back office was a harsh sentence. The following table illustrates the mismatch between Louise's talents and her tasks:

Comparison of Louise's Talent and Tasks

	Louise's Talents			Computer Job Requirements		
	High	Medium	Low	High	Medium	Low
People	x					x
Ideas	x				x	
Things			x		x	

After two years of well-paid drudgery, one fine spring morning Louise worked through a little personal analysis, gave notice on her job, accepted her first teaching position, and opened the door to career enjoyment.

A similar analysis may be helpful to you. Please use the following tables to analyze your own degree of strength in each of the three categories. Mark in each of the three—people, ideas and things—whether your preference is high, moderate, or low.

Table #3 Your Talent Table

	High	Medium	Low
Your Preferences for working with:			
People			
Ideas			
Things			

Now look back over your career patterns and analyze the requirements of at least three of the jobs you have held during your life. Choose the three in which you spent the longest number of years. What did each job require of you in terms of skills in dealing with people, aptitude for ideas, and aptitude for things (i.e. the use of your hands)?

Table #4 Part A

Analysis of The Requirements of Your Jobs

	Job #1			Job #2			Job #3		
	High	Medium	Low	High	Medium	Low	High	Medium	Low
PEOPLE									
IDEAS									
THINGS									

Have most of your jobs required the same talents? Are these the skills which are naturally yours? Please compare your analysis of your personal talents with the requirements of your career choices, and count yourself fortunate if they have matched. If your innate talents have been those which are matched by your job requirements, it is highly probable that you have already had a career marked by success and good fortune.

Paradoxically, it is these successful people who often have the most difficulty in choosing a retirement career. The person whose talents have been highly correlated with his job description is often reluctant to retire, fearful of the future, and at a loss as to what to do next. Those who have loved their work are the ones most apprehensive about leaving it. For these, retirement looms as an empty desert. Yet that desert can be made to bloom like a rose. The secret lies in designing new tasks to match your talents.

If you so far have found your jobs to be fascinating, it is a safe bet that your talents have been matched to your tasks, and that you have found yourself renewed and invigorated by your job requirements. When you choose wisely for your freedom phase, you will continue this energy and exuberance, as our many interviewees in this book can testify.

On the other hand, if you have not yet been so fortunate in your life's pathway, if your job has drained you of your energy and dusted you with defeat, this is the time for radical change. Analyze your past experiences so as to discard the boring and the exhausting. The energy you direct along the lines of your talents will produce astonishing results. The efforts channeled against the grain of your talents will leak off in random and unproductive efforts.

If your work so far has not used your major talents and tendencies you need to recognize it now and avoid doing similar work—even on a part-time basis—in your retirement years. We have a friend who has recently retired after 35 years of teaching. Although she was an excellent teacher, she always detested faculty meetings and curriculum meetings and their attendant group-think endeavors. Remembering her intolerance for these meetings, she plans in the future to avoid all committee activities and board memberships, no matter how worthy their causes, or how persuasive their membership chairmen. When she volunteers, it will be as a tutor to underprivileged children, work she can do on a one-to-one basis, and work she will thoroughly enjoy.

It will be instructive if you look again at your own employment history. This time you will need to assess it from the prospective of your likes and dislikes. Remember, you are your own authority. Your opinion is the only one that counts in this analysis. You have the right to judge and to vote, because you are designing a framework for the rest of your life. Review your employment history, beginning with your first job and going through to the present. This time, review history on a rather simplistic basis: write down what you liked the most and disliked the most about your jobs.

If you have worked for the same firm but progressed through several positions, list these positions separately:

In Table #4, Part B, list three things you liked and three things you disliked about each of the three jobs you analyzed in the preceding table.

Table #4, Part B: Position Analysis

	Position	I liked the most	I disliked the most
1. Job			
2. Job			
3. Job			

Now compare your likes from Table #4, part B with the personal talents which you listed in Table #3 and the job requirements which you listed in Table #4, part A. Can you see a pattern? Are you a people person, an idea person, a technical person, or some combination of these which is unique to you? Isn't it true that in the jobs where you have been happiest, the job requirements have been matched to your talents?

Please ask yourself two more sets of questions:

Often   Sometimes   Seldom

1. When am I a leader?
2. When am I a follower?
3. When am I a team player?
4. When am I an independent?

Even if the answers to these questions are not immediately evident, please respond to the next set:
When you are working on a project, would you rather:
a. Work alone?
b. Work from clearly outlined specifications?
c. Work as a member of a team?
d. Plan the project and leave the actual work to others?
e. Boss the job?
f. Lead the team?

Rank your answers to this set of questions and compare these answers with your responses to the four just preceding.

Finally, consider your temperament. Are you a conceptualist, one who tries to see the big picture and make sense out of life, one who is not comfortable with a project unless there is a clear vision of *how* it fits into a conceptual framework? Perhaps you are a catalyst, people-oriented, action-oriented, interested in the *who* and *what* of life. Then, again, you may be a structuralist, more comfortable with structure and responsibility than with dreaming. With this brief synthesis as a background, please analyze your future job requirements one more time.

When you are working on a project, how important are the following conditions to you? Please check how you feel about each condition:

	Essential	Desirable But Not Essential	Not Essential
Challenge			
Adventure			
Understanding the Total Picture			
Structure			
Getting Results			

The world needs all kinds of people and talents. You need to acknowledge the categories which have appeal for you, and design your retirement on the basis of this knowledge. In the chapters that follow we will develop a method of doing this.

Your retirement career change may be radical or gentle, daring or comfortable, geographic or metaphysical. But the search for a vital future begins with your acceptance of your individual responsibility for your own choices. Analyze your yesterdays, look in hope toward your tomorrows, and choose to enjoy the game of life.

CHAPTER 7
CHOOSE YOUR NEXT CAREER

"Youth is an experiment; maturity is a happy result." Anonymous

Most people have a mental list of the things they want to do when they retire. Often this list is a consensus of those things considered by the general public to be desirable—fishing, traveling, golfing, volunteering. For many, retirement becomes a quick skid into anonymity, a condition hardly designed to furnish either fun or profit to their empty days. The alternative to anonymity has its own set of barriers.

One of the first barriers we have to cross is that of relinquishing our claim on our past achievements. It is hard to come to grips with the realization that our past professional achievements no longer matter. Retirement forces us to get acquainted with our most basic selves. After the trappings and routine of our career have been left behind, we are forced to reinvent our vision of ourselves. Early retirement or forced retirement can be a blessing, because it affords the chance to face this issue abruptly, while there is still time enough to realize other dreams.

What are our remaining "duties?" We have a duty to live as long as we can, and to promote as much happiness as possible as long as we live. We have the duty to be responsible for ourselves. The reinvention of our identity, an identity separate from any other person or institution, is a project worthy of our best efforts. This reinvention provides opportunity to do our best. To prepare for individualism is to prepare to live a long time and to add life to each of your days.

After you have relinquished your claim on your past achievements, accept the fact of your own importance. This may seem to fly in the face of the advice given in an earlier paragraph, in which we urge you to re-invent your own identity. The two ideas are not in conflict, however. If your importance came from your position in your company, you may feel yourself to be stripped of your identity when you leave the company.

Your acceptance of your individual worth as a person of talent and quality is essential to your vision for your future. We are told that, "As a man thinketh in his heart, so is he." You must think of yourself as a person of importance, a person who has a contribution yet to make. Prepare to live truly, to give freely, and to define your worth, not in terms of job title or organizational chart, but in the true coin of the realm—your own character and talent.

Louise believes that it is particularly difficult for women to make choices for changing their own lives. In spite of their education, and in spite of liberation, most seek from others permission to choose change. Choosing is not easy. To choose one career or lifestyle or geographic location is to give up others. As long as we make no choice at all we can retain the illusion that all choices are possible. The danger is that these choices may be postponed too long.

Decision-making is hard. It may be harder for

women than it is for men, because often women want to please those they love more than they want to please themselves. But the requirement for choice is an essential part of the human condition.

Women now of retirement age, even though they may have chosen to have careers, were likely to have chosen that career from among the helping professions which serve the larger goals of humanity. Women who have had children usually have sublimated career to family, to balancing the precarious seesaw of love and work, attempting to please their circles of family, friends, and career. Small wonder that women are intuitive, and small wonder that many are unaccustomed to practicing the skills of rational choice in the pursuit of their own happiness. Often retirement brings their first opportunity for individual choice. Louise describes her own decisions, and her choice of a retirement pattern, as yet another turning point in a life which had already taken a good many turns:

"During the course of a twenty five year career as an educator, I made many choices, many good, some poor. I tried to learn from the poor ones and profit from the good ones, and had even taught courses about decision-making. Even so, when I was faced with the need to choose my own design for my freedom years I wished for the wisdom of Solomon and was forced to fall back on my own decidedly lesser talents. I began by facing the truth that change is inevitable. The world around us continues its relentless progress. If we refuse to change and to grow, if we indulge in unjustified complacency, the events of the world will cause our own sphere of influence to fade and shrink. We need a sense of perspective. Whole continents continue to be eroded by time and tide, and certainly the accomplishments of the fleeting careers of mere mortals are written in the shifting sands.

"I decided to take this condition of life as a challenge rather than a penalty, and to pack so much happiness into the remaining decades of my life that I would consider them to be a victory. But to do this it was necessary to choose yet another career for my retirement years. Not having given the accumulation of money a high priority, the option of spending my time primarily in volunteer work was a luxury I could not afford.

"So I went through the steps of decision strategy, asking the necessary questions in a logical sequence. I reasoned that the decision called for unflinching honesty. The time for conforming to societal expectations was long past. It was time to satisfy my own needs. I had always been somewhat out of step, anyway, and had grown accustomed to a swift pace and a fast shuffle.

"In an era when most girls when to college to major in matrimony, I earned a degree in mathematics at the age of nineteen. This was followed by marriage, a master's degree in mathematics, and a satisfying career as a statistician and college teacher. At the age of twenty eight I chose to enjoy motherhood, and with considerable efficiency produced three children in less than five years. Reentering the work force at the age of forty, I found a new career teaching mathematics in a community college, when community colleges were just beginning to change the American education scene. It was a world I loved. In a culture when the wives of most professional men did not accept paid employment, I made vague apologies for my socially peculiar propensities, and kept right on working. When I earned a Ph.D. the wife who was a working professional was still a rarity. The reputation of being different from the usual suburban wife and mother was a small price to pay for the rewards of teaching.

"I became a dean, then director of instruction of a large metropolitan community college system, and inevitably, there came a day when I faced the calendar. Never having been one who preferred to have my life's decisions made by others, I began my retirement planning by asking myself some hard questions, the same ones which are listed below."

These are the questions Louise asked:
1. What does it take to make me happy?
2. What are my strengths and skills?
3. How can these strengths and skills fit into the needs and wishes of the world around me?
4. What options can I design that combine my answers to the first three questions?
5. What is the probability of gain in each of these options?
6. What is the best option?
7. What are my strategies for success in it?

Your answer 5 which assesses the probability of gain should clearly distinguish between psychological gain (your happiness quotient) and financial gain. A rational business school approach to decision-making can be transferred into a rational approach to personal decision-making with the addition of the information gained from the consideration of your happiness quotient. After you have thoroughly examined your lists of strengths and considered different options, it is a useful devise to set up a personal decision table to assist you in your analysis.

TABLE V: DECISION TABLE

	Gains		Costs		
Options	Financial	Psychological	Financial	Psychological	Risks
Plan One					
Plan Two					
Plan Three					
Plan Four					
Plan Five					

Louise began her analysis at the age of sixty, and devised a long-term strategy to support the option which appeared best suited to her strengths. Perhaps her case will serve as an illustration of the decision-making process. First she analyzed what she had liked and disliked about her past positions. She filled out her job analysis table. These are her answers to the decision-making questions:

TABLE IV, Part B: Louise's Job Analysis

Position	Liked	Disliked
1. Oil Company Computer	1. The pay 2. Understanding the project and the computations	1. Loneliness at work 2. Not having any input into the project design 3. Routine and repetitive calculations
2. Teacher of Mathematics	1. Interacting with students 2. Lecturing and explaining 3. Actually seeing the students understanding mathematics 4. Increasing my own knowledge 5. Educational research 6. The academic environment	1. Teaching the same ideas over and over 2. Giving tests 3. Grading papers
3. Dean of Faculty	1. Prestige 2. Faculty interactions 3. Leading in curriculum 4. Chairing meetings 5. Acting as a catalyst for change 6. Public relations.	1. Building class schedules 2. Student registration 3. Working with tight budget 4. Mandatory evaluation of teachers according to rigid methodology

Then she asked and answered these questions:

Question 1: What does it take to make me happy?

Answer: Interaction with people—speaking, teaching, leading, conceptualizing, and socializing. To be absolutely honest, I am a ham and enjoy being on center stage. I like challenges, change, creative endeavors, and solving problems.

Question 2: What are my strengths and skills?

Answer:

Internal Stengths:

The ability to analyze and synthesize is perhaps my greatest strength. I believe I combine this with interpersonal skills. These skills include much experience in planning, writing, speaking, organizing, and interacting with people.

External Strengths and Experience:

a. I have a network of friends and professional associates in the national community college systems.
b. For three years I wrote a column for the newspaper in the city which was my former home. This column was a monthly feature of the editorial page.
c. I have a long history of community work, and have served on many volunteer boards.
d. I have been a pathbreaker in the world of working women.
e. I have had considerable experience in building networks, whether civic, social, or professional.

Question 3: What do I dislike?

Answer: I dislike routine, record keeping, monotony, and taking orders, I have no mechanical ability and little desire to acquire any.

Question 4: How can these strengths and skills fit into the needs and wishes of the world around me?
Answer: Working women need help in managing their lives so as to combine their careers, and the requirements of their families. I have three decades of experience in this.

My city needs an improved system of public education; I have thirty years' experience in education.

Most children need improved instruction in mathematics. I am a good mathematics teacher.

In these uncertain times many people want practical advice on career management.

The country needs good government and good schools on all levels.

Women want and need hope and inspiration.

America needs the talents of all its responsible adults—both men and women.

Question 5: What options can I design that combine my answers to the first three questions?
Answer:

Option 1 Run for public office on the local level.

Option 2 Begin a new teaching career as a substitute teacher of mathematics in the public schools.

Option 3 Based on a forty-year track record, start a speaking and seminar business advising working women.

Option 4 Forget paid work entirely, concentrate on writing, and relocate in Ireland where my fixed income would be equivalent to the cost of living.

Option 5 Found, administer, and teach in a for-profit school to teach adults the basic competencies—reading, computation, writing, communication skills.

Question 6: What is the probability of gain associated with each option?

Answer: These are displayed in the personal decision table below.

TABLE V: DECISION TABLE

Options	Gains		Costs		Risks
	Financial	Psychological	Financial	Psychological	
1. Candidate for public office	low	high	high	very high	high
2. Substitute teacher of Mathematics	low	very low	none	high	0
3. Speaker/seminar director	moderate	high	moderately low	low	mod high
4. Relocate and write	none	low	very low	high	0
5. Start prep. school	low	moderate	high	moderately high	high

Louise evaluated each option in terms of gains, costs, and risks:

1. The prospect of attaining public office on a local level offered the high psychological gains of dealing with people and issues but small financial gains. Paradoxically, the financial costs of mounting a successful campaign would be exorbitant, and these would be accompanied by the psychological uncertainties (costs) which are part and parcel of a candidate's existence. The combination of high costs, high risks, and how financial gains made this option unacceptable.

2. The option of becoming a substitute teacher of mathematics held small appeal. The current tensions inside most metropolitan public schools do little to encourage good teachers to do substitute work. This job would combine all the things Louise had disliked about teaching; while offering few of the things she had liked. The gains would be low and the psychological costs would be high. Although more acceptable than idleness, this option still holds the expectation of low gains and high stress.

3. The option of public speaking offered tempting vistas. The combination of financial gain and high psychological gain was extremely appealing. This option would mean starting her own business, with moderate costs involved. The risks were considerable. Success in this demanding profession would require most of the attributes Louise had liked about her previous jobs. Marketing would pose a considerable challenge. But to one of Louise's temperament, the challenges and the rewards far outweighed the costs. The risks would have to be managed through specific strategies.

4. The option of moving to Ireland was a fall-back position, no financial gain, low psychological gain, low financial costs, and high psychological costs occasioned by the loneliness of relocation in a completely new environment, but little or no risks.

5. An efficient adult preparatory school could be positioned in response to a large market in Louise's city. Such a school was feasible in terms of human resources and expertise. This option would require considerable capital. Start-up costs would be high, and might be disproportionate to the moderate psychological gains and low financial gains which would reasonably be expected. Such a school would

fill a definite need. But the administration position would emphasize all the things Louise had disliked about being an administrator—tight budget, teacher evaluation, efficient class scheduling.

Question 5: What is the probability of gain in each option?

Three of the options showed promise of gain: public office, public speaking, and adult school administration and teaching. All three were risky ventures; two of the three were high cost ventures. The other two options, substitute mathematics teacher, and relocating to Ireland, were risk-free, but carried little expectation of gain, either financial or psychological.

Question 6: What is the best option?

For one with Louise's likes and dislikes, and her extroverted and risk-taking temperament, the option of becoming a public speaker and seminar leader was the best. Combining expectations of moderate financial gains with high psychological gains and moderately low start-up costs, it offered the best expectation. Louise chose this option and began the design of a long-range strategy.

Question 7: What are the associated strategies?

Answer: A pathbreaker in the field of working women, Louise had enjoyed decades of work in male-dominated professions. She concluded that it was insufficient merely to have been successful in these careers; credibility often rests most readily on tangible evidence. So she wrote a book on career decision-making for women, and used the book as a booster to launch a part-time speaking career. Concurrently she polished her skills and earned references by giving free speeches at local conferences and seminars. The combination proved to be an effective first-stage booster. Hard work and high enthusiasm are an effective combination in most ventures. Louise felt that she would not truly develop into her own true self until she had tested whether or not she could compete successfully outside an institutional environment. She was eager to test her wings as an entrepreneur. Encouraged by her friends and emboldened by beginning successes, she planned for a major change. The next requirements were optimistic expectations and perseverance.

To glimpse the possibility of success is miraculously revitalizing. Many people experience a slump in their middle years, when life becomes routine and wearing. The design of a new business or the creation of a new work of art, or the use of a neglected talent, will bring on new energy. As your own project becomes reality you will experience a burst of creativity and enthusiasm. When you honestly believe that the remaining distance to your goal is short, this newly generated energy will carry you forward to success.

Many who retire from major corporations or institutions will experience major changes in attitude in their freedom years. Even those who prided themselves on the efficiency with which they advanced their corporate goals will find their lives in their freedom years to be happier than ever before. The difference lies in the act of creation. If you have designed your own business, or service, or work of art, you can take justifiable and personal pride from its successful completion. It is human nature to try harder where much is at stake. Your margin of success will be defined by that willingness to try harder. Paradoxically, this extra work will lead not to exhaustion but exhilaration. You will be renewed by your efforts even as you are rewarded by your successes.

CHAPTER 8
REACH YOUR FULL POTENTIAL

"The secret of happiness is freedom and the secret of freedom is a brave heart." Pericles

A wise man once defined success as living the kind of life you WANT to live and becoming the kind of person you want to become. This does not come about through magic, but through progressive steps toward an understood and predefined goal. A successful life under the right circumstances is an easy and natural existence, and for a fortunate few this is indeed possible. For most of us, however, success depends on discipline and continual progress toward the goals we have mapped out for ourselves. Success begins with the creation within each of us of those qualities which generate success.

In this chapter we shall take an imaginary journey. Three bridges must be crossed. Each will bring us closer to our goal of a happy and successful life. There is no shortcut to reach the goal. Each of us must travel the highway that leads over all three bridges.

Do not be misled into impatience. The speed of your progress is secondary. Of major importance is the direction of your route. Have patience, keep sight of your goals, and do not be led astray into detours. Patience is not an easy virtue, but there is no quick route to success. People do not explode into success. They grow into it.

And now for the journey across the three bridges. None of the crossings is easy. You must develop certain strengths for each bridge, and new strengths are required for each crossing. But you will grow strong on the journey.

The first and most essential bridge is one that most are loathe to admit ever exists. This is the connecting link between FEAR and COURAGE. It is the most important step in your journey. You must prepare for it by realizing that it is normal to feel fear and apprehension.

Nature has provided us with the quality of fear as a part of our instinct for self-preservation. But how do we deal with it? First, you should meet this problem on the basis that courage is not overcoming fear; rather, it is standing our ground in spite of it. It is no disgrace to be afraid—the disgrace is in refusing to rise above fear. No one has ever failed because he was afraid. He who fails does so because he fails to rise above his fear. We should never wish to remove the butterflies from our stomachs: we only want to teach them to fly in formation.

So how do we meet the problem of fear? First, we accept the fact that fear is born of uncertainty and lack of knowledge. Sam was afraid when his hog farm was faced with economic debt, and he was afraid because the forces causing this terrible turn of events seemed beyond his control. We are afraid when we are confronted with the need for our own development. We fear what we do not understand. We fear that which is unfamiliar: we fear that which we need to learn. For Sam, the unforeseen loss of his way of life as well as his livelihood forced the need for major change. To be thrust into relearning and retraining at the end of a highly successful career would have devastated many men. But Sam had courage.

It is a rule of life that advancement carries the price tag of anxiety. Its corollary is that avoidance of anxiety is a road that leads to obscurity, the road that cowards take.

It is logical, therefore, that to rise above fear, we should learn the maximum about the factor that causes anxiety. Whether selling a product, trying a case, running for office, raising a child, or preparing for another career, it is all the same. We do not have the courage that enables us to overcome fear and speak with authority until we know what we are doing.

Sam set out to learn all he could about the profession he wished to enter. He knew that making music was not enough, that liking people was not enough. Success in his newly chosen profession would have to be preceded by learning all he could about the process of teaching. With the help of an enthusiastic academic advisor at the state university, Sam immersed himself in a course of study that was remarkable for its intensity. Others might have been afraid to enter into competition with fellow students younger than his own sons. Sam had the courage of his convictions. He was rewarded with the confidence that comes from earned accomplishment. And he learned that the joy of learning need not be confined to the young.

Sam was determined to gain an understanding of the theory behind the practice of music. He knew that we must know the reasons behind our actions. An intelligent man seasoned in the school of life, Sam knew that we must know the why behind the what to be truly qualified to deal successfully with the task of teaching others. His fear had arisen from lack of knowledge about this future. Courage flowed to him as he gained knowledge about his new profession.

But knowledge and certainty, important as they are, are alone not enough to carry us across the bridge to courage and determination. The next bridge is crossed through belief. Every law of physics has a corresponding mental and emotional law. Newton tells us that for every force there must be an opposing and equal force. The emotional corollary is that fear, to be successfully opposed, must be counter-balanced by an equal emotion. This counter-balance is knowledge and understanding. They will provide the opposite and equal force, and even tip the balance positively toward belief. When Sam had completed his course of study, completing a three-year program in two years, his optimistic plans for the future were grounded in belief. He was ready to persuade others that he was ready to enter a new profession. Persuading others is merely the act of converting people to our way of believing. Unless we have sincere belief and deep conviction, there is, in reality, nothing to which we can convert people. Knowledge is the key to a new career, but belief unlocks the door at the job interview.

The essence of salesmanship is the knowledge that people are not convinced by the power of logic. They are convinced by the depth of our conviction—by our belief. We are converted by the deep and sincere conviction that we ourselves believe, deeply and truly, in the worth of our endeavor. So fear is displaced by knowledge, which leads to courage. Belief is the bridge that leads to confidence and experience.

Courage is a state of mind. Confidence is a state of being. This transition is a conditioning process rather than a learning process. It is perfected by doing, rather than knowing. In other words, knowledge must be followed by experience. A person must be knowledgeable and enthusiastic in order to have courage, but he must accomplish an experience in order to have confidence.

Sam moved into his teaching career with the confidence of a born winner. He drew on the memories of his many successes during his decades as a hog farmer: he knew himself to be astute, energetic, knowledgeable. He knew that he had superb people skills. He refused to let the memory of his bankruptcy haunt his days or limit his vision of the future. And the people of his community concurred. Far from being regarded as a failure, Sam is regarded by his students and his peers as a successful man. He is successful at the business of life.

Sam's confidence grows with accomplishments. Results increase his confidence. The sure knowledge that he has succeeded in the past and will undoubtedly continue to succeed in the future is the bridge that transports him from courage to confidence. The same can be true for you.

As you cross this second bridge of belief your doubts will be removed and your fears laid to rest. Your approach to future plans will no longer be based on hope and speculation but on the sweet remembrance of past successes. Certainty comes from the sure knowledge of previous accomplishments. Hope is ephemeral; knowledge and confidence lift toward a new realm, a new plateau of accomplishment. As true today as it was for the Romans, the basis for the success of Caesar's armies was succinctly told by Cicero: *Posse quid possum obdent* "They can because they KNOW they can."

Confidence and certainty are two of the most powerful weapons in your arsenal. Nothing is better. The world makes way for the person who acts as though he knows where he is going. It was true at the time of Caesar, true for our pioneering ancestors, and will prove equally valid for you.

When experience has provided you with a solid track record of accomplishments and the confidence that comes from progress, you will approach the third and final bridge. This bridge will carry you from the land of confidence into the green pastures of freedom. Never easily available, and appreciated the more because of the obstacles which have impeded its pathway, Freedom carries with it a risk which must be knowledged and withstood.

There is a recognized hazard which is the price of success. The great industrialist, Charles F. Kettering, often said, "Do not bring me your successes, they weaken me; bring me your failures, they strengthen me." Too frequently, success lends itself to the seduction of ease and idleness, causing the unwary to discard the very qualities which made freedom possible.

There is an old saying, "If you want to destroy a person, give him too much too soon." History is punctuated by examples of people who reached the top through hard work and sacrifice, only to succumb to the temptations which are all too available to the successful. Beware lest yesterday's laurels become tomorrow's goals. Past accomplishments, rather than becoming a challenge to future achievement, often become an excuse for present failure. Worse yet, they can become the unhealthy axis around which the rest of our life revolve.

Any person who selects a goal which can be readily achieved has defined his own limitations. When we cease to grow we begin to die. Tennyson expresses the idea in the wandering of Ulysses, "I am a part of all that I have met; yet all experience is an arch where through gleams that untraveled world whose margin fades forever and forever as I move."

It is one of the blessings of life that we continually travel toward an ever-beckoning horizon. Fortunate is the person whose reach exceeds his grasp.

Freedom brings happiness and is the victory not easily attained. And even when victory has been achieved it must be won over and over again. it is not easy to have hitched one's wagon to a star, but the very difficulty of the journey adds zest. The opportunities of life create their own excitement. The rewards of freedom belong to the brave and courageous, those who dare, and dream, and aim for the best.

The story of Harlan Sanders can serve as a lesson to us all. Sanders, who is known to the world as Colonel Sanders, the founder of Kentucky Fried Chicken, was not born with a silver spoon in his mouth. In fact, as a child he was lucky to have a spoon in his mouth at all. His father died when he was six. By the age of seven he was the family cook, for his mother worked long hours outside the home in order to feed her children. This grim childhood instilled in Harlan Sanders a lifelong respect for hard work; along with this respect came a trait more rare—he loved to work. Embracing necessity, he enjoyed work, hated vice, was suspicious of welfare, and even as a child grew into self-reliance.

He had ample opportunity to practice his beliefs. Entirely self-reliant by the age of 15, his formal education ended at the seventh grade. Yet his respect for learning would not be denied, and he took a correspondence course in law which enabled him to function in Justice of the Peace courts in the south. For twenty-five years he held a series of varied and poorly-paid jobs. Finally, he believed himself to be in sight of success. He became a business owner operating a cafe in Corbin, Kentucky. His specialty, Kentucky Fried Chicken, enjoyed a substantial and loyal following of customers from the area. Had he not met with an unexpectedly harsh turn of events he might well have remained a local businessman, counting his life to have been modestly successful.

Fate ruled otherwise. At the age of 65 Sanders' business was wiped out when the new interstate highway by-passed his cafe. A man less tempered by adversity would have cursed fate and quit. But at the age of 66, Harlan Sanders set out with his pressure cooker and his special seasonings to sell his secret and establish a fried chicken franchise business. He set his sights on building his dream. The rest is legend. The franchise company which he founded in 1956 with faith, and grit, and a handful of spices became a multi-million dollar operation. Although the colonel sold the business for two million dollars in 1964, it has gone on to make millionaires out of more than 100 people since that time.

Colonel Sanders based his success on his own talents. In spite of his modest beginnings, these were not modest talents, nor did he have any patience with modest efforts. To the end of his long life he preached and practiced the love of work and the dedication to extra effort which were at the central core of his character. In being true to himself he lived his dream. No doubt it was all the sweeter for having been begun at the age of sixty-six.

It would be an injustice to portray the journey from fear to courage, from courage to confidence, and from confidence to freedom as being a path of roses. It is a pilgrim's road, full of obstacles and sacrifices. But the promise of strength is implicit in the hazards of the journey. We can say of this pilgrim as the Californians say of the "Forty-Niners": "The west was won by the strong and hardy. The cowards never left home, the weak died along the way, and only the strong survived to settle California."

True success lies in the conduct of the journey of life, and not necessarily in its ultimate end. This is illustrated in a beautiful story related to us by a world traveler.

Said he, "I once had an unusual experience in my travels abroad. I saw a flock of lowland butterflies caught in some strange migratory impulse, flying steadfastly for great mountains, far above their natural home. In the desperately cold and thinning air of the Himalayan snow, they fell, one by one. But every butterfly was still headed indomitably for the high peaks, and each struggling set of wings beat bravely, even unto death itself."

The human race advances only through the achievements of the individual. May we each live so as to accept our portion of responsibility for this advancement, and may we remain true to this vision as long as we live.

CHAPTER 9
FLOURISH IN ADVERSITY

"The days that are still to come are the wisest witnesses." Pindar

Most of us are already familiar with adversity. Children of the Depression, adults during World War II, we are not strangers to hardship. But how many of us have come to regard adversity as the friend it can be? There is a picture which vividly portrays this powerful thought. Protruding from a dead stump, a green and healthy branch is living and growing. Just beneath the picture is the word, *Reviresco*. The liberal translation is, "I flourish in adversity." How fortunate you are if you have already learned that we grow strong only through adversity.

Obstacles give to life the strength that carbon gives to steel. "Hardships," as Lincoln expressed it, "are too precious to lose." Although the tempering we receive through the hardships of our pasts may not have been appreciated at the time, if we learned and grew from the experiences, as many of us did, we have an inestimable advantage over those whose lives have lacked this tempering. This advantage will become apparent as you plan for your next career.

It may be true that life is a grindstone, but it is equally true that whether it grinds us or polishes us is determined by the substance of which we are made. An event considered by one person to be misfortune may be viewed by another as a great adventure. The stumbling block to the timid is a stepping stone to the one who is more courageous. Most have already been handed an occasional lemon by life—the optimistic ones have already learned the art of turning it into lemonade. You have already had the advantage of learning how to earn a living, of learning to be self reliant, of learning how to stand on your own feet. Far better than those younger than you, you already know the relationship between making money and the joy of spending it. Standards of performance in this competitive world are getting higher and higher. You will have a definite advantage, the advantage of being tempered by adversity.

In the past few years in this country the story has been repeated all too frequently. A company finds itself forced to close its doors, or to cut back its production so drastically that massive lay-offs are inevitable. In many cases the newspaper headlines are quickly translated into personal tragedies. The man or woman who is faced with the loss of a job after decades of employment is suddenly plunged into despair. Anger and resentment are swiftly followed by a humiliating anxiety. Yet, for many, the situation turns out to be a blessing in disguise.

The anxiety comes from being dependent on another's decision, trained by a lifetime's habits of employment in and loyalty to some other person's company. The price of the comfort of letting yourself be kept in the employment of another is, in the end, an awful insecurity. There is a numbing insecurity when a company fails and its people are flung out unprotected into the jobless cold.

Many find that leaving their company after decades of association is as jolting as leaving a family. It is well to realize that the degrees of allegiance are decidedly different. The ties of blood are lasting; we belong to our families for all of our lives. Companies, on the other hand, can sever the association with startling efficiency and finality. Companies are legal organizations, not emotional holding patterns, and certainly not families. The person who assumes otherwise is apt to be in for a rude awakening. The analogy is not to be found in human relationships: the person who faces forced retirement is in the position of the bird which has been kicked out of the nest. The nest may have been soft, it may have been high—it may even have been famous—but it is no longer available as an option.

Small wonder that many face the prospect of their leave-taking with apprehension. But the prospect of flying offers vistas that can never be seen from the nest. Twenty to thirty years in the structured environment of corporate or institutional worlds serve as an inhibiting preparation for freedom. Some who have spent their careers in such environments find themselves unprepared to flap their wings, and worse, philosophically opposed to the need for doing it. They flutter around in the cold, half-heartedly flapping their wings and seeking another warm nest. Others conquer their fears and begin their flight training. But we are not permanently entitled to the structure of the encompassing nest; structure imposed by our first career can be unlearned. We can learn to love freedom, and rejoice in its opportunities.

Emerson said, "Our strength grows out of our weakness. When we are pricked and stung and sorely shot at, then there is awakened in us the indignation that arms itself with secret force. A great man is always willing to be little. While he sits on the cushion of advantages he goes to sleep. When he is pushed, tormented, and defeated he has a chance to learn something."

Every adversity has within it the seeds of opportunity. There is a certain dignity in the human spirit which always becomes more clearly visible during the moment which threatens defeat.

It takes a real man to be improved by defeat, and we interviewed one who serves as a role model for many. Don Fambrough is an impressive man. The first impression is one of strength: physical strength, moral strength, intellectual strength. Don Fambrough is not a lightweight. His strengths are those developed when a man of character is repeatedly tested in the crucible of life.

It hurts to get fired. It hurts more to get fired in the spotlight. But to have earned the dubious distinction of being the only head football coach in the nation to have been fired TWICE by the same university is more than a good coach deserves. A man who has twice been through the public pain of a high-voltage dismissal has had his full share of adversity, measured out, pressed down, and running over.

Even so, if he had it all to do over again, Don would choose challenge and change over boredom. There is no doubt in his mind that the shining hours more than make up for the hard times.

Don has never yet had a morning when he hated to go to work. He felt that way about coaching, and he feels the same way about his present work. He loves people, he loves his work, and he loves football.

As a boy growing up on a Texas ranch he got home training in fortitude. With colts and calves as playmates and three pine poles for a goal post, he started his own early training in football. But the solitude of the ranch was temporary. He spent his adult life surrounded by people. A high school football star, a scholarship student at the University of Texas, after World War II, Don transferred to the University of Kansas and found his true home. He has given it his deep and abiding loyalty ever since.

Don dislikes boredom and he dislikes losing. The combination has kept him a busy and happy man for most of his life. What he enjoys is continued excitement. For thirty five years football was his life—through good times and bad times—seven days a week, twelve months a year.

At the core of his being is his relationship with his family. His boys became his extended family. As a coach, he became their adopted father. They worked together, dreamed together, suffered together, and rejoiced together. He taught each boy the joy of playing his heart out, the joy of creative expectancy.

So deep is Don's commitment to the University of Kansas that when he was fired as head coach for the first time, he publicly stated that he would never coach against the university. He stayed on in the athletic department, preparing to give his full measure of effort in any capacity that would contribute to the school. By the time he was hired again and fired again, he had been with the university for thirty five years. This time he felt the totality of the situation—a total emptiness, a total silence. It was time to come to terms with the rest of his life.

When all his extraneous emotions had been burned

away, it was his family and his loyalty that formed the ground of his being. From that ground he built a new life, faced his grief, and worked through it.

Don knew that he knew how to coach. He wondered whether he was capable of doing anything else. He felt like football had wired him, inspired him, hired him, and fired him. As it has turned out, his new career has revived him.

For the past four years, Don Fambrough has been a field representative for the senior senator from Kansas. His talents redirected, he now deals with the problems of people all over the state. His skill in understanding and interpreting their problems to the senator is of vital importance. Don has found a new life, and in this new career he has found that football does not have a monopoly on problems. He is working now in a larger arena.

He travels the state of Kansas two to three days a week. Advance press releases inform the senator's constituents of Don's schedule. After thirty five years of recruiting, Don knows the state like the back of his hand. He knows its people, they are tremendously important to him, and they have confidence in him.

Each morning he feels like it is just before the kickoff. Wherever he goes he deals with the human conditions of hardship and hope, problems and solutions, working and winning. To Don, the game of life is endlessly fascinating. He is now in a whole new world.

His is an attitude of optimism. He believes the people in this country are getting a grip on reality, combining the time-tested arts of good management and efficiency with the knowledge afforded by a new age of technology. He believes that the beleagured farmers who are the senator's constituents will emerge as winners. And he cares about their winning their economic struggles with the same intensity that he once directed toward winning football games.

His advice to others is succinct, "Life does not end when you are fired and life does not end when you are retired. Get off your duff and go for it!"

We count Don to be a truly successful man. Along with his physical travels, he is a man on a metaphysical highway, journeying the road to suigeneris.

For many facing retirement and the design of a new career, the adversity may be financial. Particularly this is true for women. Women now facing retirement have earned substantially less money than men during their salaried years. Consequently, their pensions and their Social Security benefits are all too frequently far less than those of the men who are their contemporaries. In contrast, women can expect to live much longer. It takes but the most elementary knowledge of arithmetic to conclude that many women in retirement will need to figure out a method to supplement their income.

But success and failure constitute a two-edged sword. Just as we attain success by making ourselves vulnerable to failure, so we can experience the joys of life only by being willing to expose ourselves to the pains and sufferings of existence. Many women will freely admit they have had both. This openness to life, this willingness to experience it all, leads to a strength of character which can lend zest to the freedom phase of life.

We believe that the woman who expects to carve a new life out of her retirement years has, perhaps for the first time in her life, exactly the same chance for economic success as does a man. Success in the future will depend not on physical strength but on the qualities of people skills and of communication skills, the ability to persuade others, the ability to intuitively decide how to best serve others, the ability to reason, and the willingness to work. Women through the ages have had reason to master these skills. In the service economy which will be America's primary economic base during the next few years, women of maturity and vision will have unprecedented opportunities.

We like the sentiment in a cartoon which shows a tall wall with the shining sun giving generously of its beams on one side. On the other side were only shadows. Where the sun had shown at the base of the wall there were a number of small flowers. On the shady side there was one giant flower whose head was above the wall. Underneath the drawing were these few lines: "How great this shaded plant has grown, how tall. Her sisters on the sunny side are neither tall nor high; but this one had to reach for light or die."

If you are a woman preparing for retirement, you may be facing your first opportunity to reach for the sun. Go for it! Do not be held back by the platitudes of your more timid contemporaries nor the assumptions that were appropriate to generations past. The rules which worked for your mother and grandmother are likely to be of little good to you. Accept the joys and responsibilities of becoming a pathfinder. Look for the path that belongs to you.

We recently interviewed a woman who served as a wonderful example. Betty moved briskly in the arctic air as she packed her car on a Sunday afternoon, preparing for her usual week on the road as a public relations representative. The emergency kit was the first item she packed, a necessity for a woman traveling alone on the January roads of the west. She hummed a little tune, already reviewing in her mind the nursing homes she would visit as a representative of a large company which owns and operates thirty-three nursing homes in a three-state territory.

A trim, sweet-faced woman, her sixty two years sit lightly on Betty. In fact, they sit so lightly that when we interviewed her she had to pause and think to remember her calendar age. But this attitude is a relatively recent achievement. Ten years ago, Betty felt herself to be old, a defeated woman with a bleak future. Yet another habitual victim of a wife-battering husband, she lived a life of quiet tragedy, in dread of her present and afraid of her future.

Betty can identify the moment which was an inflection point in her life, the moment her life changed direction. She was lying in bed in a motel room on the rainy Sunday morning following her mother's funeral. Enveloped by a despondency which went far beyond her grief for the loss of her beloved mother, she remembers thinking that she wished that she would never have to get out of bed again. Then one of her grandchildren turned on the television set, and she heard Dr. Robert Schuller, the evangelist, saying to her, "This is the day that the Lord hath made. Rejoice and be exceedingly glad!" The words seemed to be spoken directly to her. She felt herself being turned toward an affirmation of life, and she feels that this help and support came at the time of a turning point in her life. Dr. Schuller's books and television sermons reached out to her in a way which enabled her to make the difficult decisions necessary to change the patterns of her life.

She told us that all her subsequent hardships were endured with a faith in God and an assurance in His love.

From this inner conviction, this necessity for courage, Betty finally did summon the will to leave her marriage. Following a carefully-constructed plan, she slipped away in the night to a temporarily safe haven. There followed recriminations, a bitter court battle, and then years of poverty, hardship, and self-doubt.

When Betty left her role as a middle-class housewife she began a precarious existence. She became a student in a community college, bussing tables in the college cafeteria to earn her keep. In those troubled days she was beset by doubt, bolstered by hope, mentored by adversity. Gradually, these tremendous forces began their magic work. Betty's mental outlook shifted. Rather than considering herself to be martyr, a victim of undeserved tragedy, she began to regard herself as a woman destined to triumph over adversity. She stopped crying and began making decisions.

Soon she was offered a position as secretary to a college administrator. Again, opportunity brought the need for growth, so she resumed the course work which would form the basis for an associate degree.

As it turned out, she was still not immunized against adversity. A series of staff cutbacks eliminated her job, placing her once again on the threshold of a bleak future. This time Betty's reaction was decidedly different. This time she was angry. It was her anger that propelled her transfer to another college and to another field of study, and in this new beginning she chose a field well suited to her talents. She earned an associate degree in gerontology, gained experience as a volunteer with the United Way and the Department of Aging, and had the affirming experience of being offered her dream job.

Now in her fifth year with her employer, she has the air of confidence which comes from earned success. She travels a three-state area, speaking, selling, comforting, and loving her clients. To learn the speaking skills so necessary to her position, she joined Toastmasters, knowing that she needed both skill and confidence. Her experiences there have found their way into the tales of Toastmasters. So far as she knows, Betty is the only person to have begun her Toastmasters experience by fainting at the podium. From this inauspicious beginning she has gone forward with her customary persistence, and has recently completed her credits for the Distinguished Toastmaster Award.

Although we come to success through many doors, surely that of adversity is the most forbidding. Yet the door opened by adversity may afford us the most permanent passage, for its training provides unforgettable lessons. Betty is a late bloomer—not a rose, whose delicate petals fall early; but an aster, that hardy flower that blooms late, keeps its color, holds its petals, and will even retain its graceful beauty in dried bouquets.

As you assess the road of your future, do not be misguided by the platitudes developed for the multitude. You are not too old to change, to grow, and to rejoice in the process. Louise earned her Ph.D. at age fifty, and made a major career advancement in her late fifties, changing her city, her employer, and her job description. You may wish to design drastic measures into your future, or you may decide to create a career that will be destined for success because it utilizes your unique talents in such a way that success seems destined from the outset. Whatever you decide, do not let age nor sex deter you. Grandma Moses became famous as much for her youthful spirit as for her remarkable paintings, because that spirit was translated through every stroke of her brush.

There is the beautiful story of the wise old man who lived many centuries ago. Each day he would appear in the town square and speak words of wisdom to those who would listen. He was resented by the younger men, and they used every method to discredit him. Finally one of them called the others together and proposed a plan to run the sage out of town.

"We shall call all the townspeople together tomorrow," he said. "I shall have a bird in my hand and I shall ask the old man whether it is dead or alive. If he says it is alive I shall crush it. If he says it is dead I shall let it fly away into the sky. In either event we shall be able to turn the people against him. We shall stone him and run him out of town."

The next day the young men proceeded as they had planned. The entire village was called together and the leader began to scoff at the old man. "Old man," he said, "If you are so wise, tell me, is this bird in my hand dead or alive?"

The seer of many years paused for a moment, looked at the puzzled crowd, and then at the young men eager to witness his destruction. Finally he smiled and said softly and gently to the leader, "As thou wilt, my son, as thou wilt."

We ourselves hold our future in our own hands. It is within our power to destroy it or to let it soar. The strange thing about it is that if we look for ways to avoid meeting difficulty and obstacles, if we always seek safety—we have planted the seed of failure and it is certain to sprout. But if we gladly encounter the difficulties of life and seek to strengthen ourselves, we cannot be defeated. Regardless of your past obstacles, the future can be what you wish it to be. Aldous Huxley said, "The genius of life is carrying the spirit of childhood into old age."

Optimism allows us to triumph over adversity, persevere over troubles, and, finally, to increase our margin of success. It all boils down to the optimistic expectation that motivates us to keep trying.

The difference between success and failure is often determined by your willingness to keep on trying. We learned in physics that water boils at 212 degrees Fahrenheit, giving off steam, a great source of power. Water at 211 degrees is only hot water. Adding just one more degree of heat transforms this hot water into a mighty force. One more degree, less than one-half of one percent more heat, changes H_2O into a dynamic power that generates the electricity to provide the life pulse of great cities and turn the wheels of industry.

Consider the small statistical difference between a baseball player who bats .250 and one who bats .350. In practice, the difference is that the player with the .350 batting average gets one more hit each ten times at bat. A small statistical margin, but what a great difference! One authority states that nine out of ten players, either "out" or "safe" at first base, are "out" or "safe" by a margin of only six inches.

A certain man in Arizona spent many years prospecting for silver, looking for one of the rich silver veins near Tombstone. In one instance he ran a tunnel several hundred feet into the side of a small mountain. In discouragement, he abandoned the project and died a defeated man. Some years later a mining company was organized to buy up some of the mineral claims in the Tombstone area. One of their first projects was the extension of the old prospector's mining shaft. Less than two feet from the exact point where the old miner had stopped digging was found the second richest silver strike ever made in that area. Two feet of margin made the difference of millions of dollars.

The slender amount which differentiates force from inertia, action from inaction, success from failure, is even more profound in people. The margin which separates us from the realization of our dreams and hopes is small—sometimes tragically so.

Because the margin is so thin, the distance so short, we should all feel the challenge to try harder. To travel nine-tenths of the journey and then give up the trip is not logical. Your challenge will be to try harder in the ventures of your freedom years. If you have designed a business opportunity which is matched to your talents, if you have acquired the knowledge and the confidence born of accomplishment, then persevere in your efforts. To approach the doors of opportunity and give up on the doorstep is to sell yourself short.

Most of us, if we have the discipline to do so, can improve every phase of our lives by at least ten percent. This is more than is required for success in most endeavors. And the wonderful thing about this improvement is that we are not required to reach out for new qualities. We have only to stir up the talents that are already there.

CHAPTER 10
FIND LIFE AFTER LAY-OFF

Phoenix: A mythical bird of great beauty...fabled to live 500 years..., to burn itself on a funeral pyre, and to rise from its ashes in the freshness of youth. A person or thing that has become renewed or restored after suffering calamity.
THE RANDOM HOUSE DICTIONARY

Since 1985, approximately half a million midmanagers have been let go in this country. Much of this paring down of the administrative ranks has been brought on by the restructuring of the American economy, as the country moves from an industrial to an information nation. Part of the reduction is due to automation, as machines assume the burden of keeping track of people and material. Often these forces are felt most keenly by the thousands of middle-aged managers who have lost their corporate connections through staff reductions. Too young to quit work and too old to begin again at the bottom, many feel the keen sting of personal rejections. They are naturally apprehensive about starting over. Can old dogs really be taught new tricks? It depends on the dog.

For those with the right temperament and talent, a happy alternative has emerged. Rather than trying to re-enter the corporate world as managers—the career equivalent of beating a dead horse—some are dusting off their degrees, going back to college, and studying to become high school mathematics and science teachers. Some corporations are actually providing funding for out-placement through university teacher training programs. The Chevron Corporation, with the University of Houston, the University of New Orleans, and San Francisco State University, has designed ENCORE, a collaborative program to supply the public schools with much needed mathematics and physical science teachers.

ENCORE is the joining of two mis-matches: there are too many good people in the oil business and not enough good people in the teaching business. The shortage of qualified mathematics and science teachers in the public schools has for decades adversely affected education. The economic depression in the oilpatch may prove to be the educational equivalent of the ill-wind theory. Chevron's ENCORE program may very well prove to be a dramatic solution to this particular educational problem. Certainly it promises to boost education in its three geographic target areas.

The University of Houston takes justifiable pride in its ENCORE program, which not only trains teachers but matches them with school districts needing staff. In a brochure advertising the program, the educational requirements are clearly specified:

> A special curriculum designed to provide all of the requirements leading to the Texas Teacher's Certificate was initiated especially for this program. A natural support system among students is fostered through courses arranged exclusively for them. The three-phase program emphasizes reflective inquiry and the translation of life experiences to teaching competence.

In the first phase of their program, students are involved in two classes which introduce them to teaching. Each student spends approximately 50 hours observing, tutoring, and assisting in two local school settings.

In the second phase of the program, students focus more specifically on methods of teaching science or mathematics. Videotaped microteaching experiences give them opportunities to practice and analyze the methodologies they are learning. Principles of learning and the influence of societal trends on teaching are incorporated in the program.

University faculty are working individually as mentors with ENCORE students. They work with ENCORE students to complete program requirements and are available to discuss ideas, feelings, and concerns related to becoming a teacher.

Student teaching is the third and final phase of the program. Students complete a 12-week full-time internship under the direct supervision of their school based teacher education.

We visited Dr. John Creswell's class, where nine students were completing the requirements of the second phase of the program, learning specific methods of teaching science and mathematics. Louise, a former mathematics teacher, looked on Creswell's class as a teacher's dream come true. She saw a small group of bright and eager students, all intellectually engaged in the subject matter, all acutely attuned to each pronouncement of their professor. Cavett looked at the group from the perspective of a professional public speaker, and saw seasoned presenters who were enthusiastic and knowledgeable. We believe that these retrained professionals, already armed with first class scientific educations, can become a formidable force in the world of education.

The nine people we met have already been tested in an unsparing laboratory, the school of real life. They know first hand the qualifications required for material success. They know what it feels like to win, to rise high on the dual ladders of merit and materialism. More recently, they have learned what it feels like to lose and to be pushed off the ladder.

For most of the class, the ENCORE program will prove to be a trampoline rather than a safety net. Teaching may allow them to spring back from rejection to new heights of personal satisfaction. For a few, ENCORE may indeed be no more than a safety net, an assurance of a soft landing at the lower end of the pay scale.

Is it possible to predict these landings, to distinguish the trampoline performers from those headed for the safety net? The answers may lie in attitudes, both individual and collective. It may be that in the art and science of education, attitudes are more important than the facts. What are the distinguishing marks? How can success be predicted?

The class in itself was unusual. Each person was intelligent, motivated, and well-educated. Their backgrounds included expertise in subjects generally considered to be extremely difficult—chemistry, mathematics, physics, engineering, computer programming, geology. All brought remarkable intellectual foundations to their class in classroom methods. All brought a visual and logical approach to academic concepts. We enjoyed Waldo Gullickson's witty mini-lecture on the application of Pascal's triangle to branching theory, a lecture entitled, "Do these branches leaf you out?" Gullickson's presentation completely involved his audience, and each student obviously had the ability to become individually intrigued with the subject matter. There was no question as to the academic expertise of these would-be teachers. Academic expertise, however, is a necessary but insufficient requirement for successful teaching.

Three essential questions remain. Can these scientists communicate their own academic excitement, and succeed in intriguing their young students? If they are successful in intriguing their students, will the success of outsiders be tolerated by the current educational system? And, finally, are parents ready for teaching which emphasizes academic expertise, rigor, and hard work rather than socialization? These are not insignificant questions. The future of American education may rest on the answers.

What are the attitudes of the nine neophyte teachers? Most are living with a high degree of emotional uncertainty. This uncertainty, mixed with the proportions of hope, optimism, pessimism, enthusiasm and apprehension generated by the events of any specific day, charts an erratic emotional pattern on the daily record of their lives. All agree that the outcomes of their next semester of practice teaching will most likely tell the tale.

So far, their responses have been as varied as their lives. Their ages range from the early thirties to the mid sixties. To a degree, their responses are a function of age, but only to a degree. The sixty five year old, secure on a substantial income, dreams of repaying to the world the opportunities he has enjoyed. Another man in his fifties, knowing in his heart that he is a born teacher, ponders how best to direct his talents so as to achieve the optimum good. Still another, formerly idealistic and hopeful, has been so disillusioned with his brief periods of observation in the reality of inner city classrooms that he despairs that one man can make a difference. All are fueled by optimism, chilled by a perception of societal apathy, and anxious about their individual solutions to a major problem.

These scientists turned teachers are not representative of the population as a whole. Less than one percent of retirees will go into teaching, and even fewer will teach mathematics and science. But these nine people share an experience in common with a much larger segment of American society. All were involuntarily released from their jobs, and all went through the five stages of career death: denial, fear, anger, bargaining, acceptance. They have been fired in the crucible of a harsh economic furnace. As they sifted through the ashes of their careers, they determined that the essential matter of their character and talents would not be destroyed, but only transformed. The question remaining in each mind is whether the art and science of teaching will provide them with wings to soar above the ashes. Each hopes that teaching will become his personal phoenix.

For at least two, the question is close to being answered. For these, the inflection point which ended the downward turn of their careers and marked the upward direction of their new hopes has already appeared. Two of the students have already been offered teaching positions and are excited about their choices.

For one of these men, the new opportunity has already forced the confrontation of a new dilemma: should he accept the plum job of teaching university-bound juniors and seniors in an honors program at a magnet high school? Or should he focus his efforts on teaching the concepts of science to impressionable fifth and sixth graders in the hopes of making a difference in the lives of the underprivileged? His personal philosophy of education is being forged as he wrestles with this choice. But his win/win option has as yet not been extended to his class mates.

Another, with a brilliant record and a masters degree in chemistry from Oxford University, in England, fears that he is regarded by the educational establishment as being over-qualified. He wonders whether his past achievements may bar his acceptance by the teaching professionals who make up the school's search committees. His task may be to get hired in spite of his record.

Newcomers without degrees from colleges of education face real opposition from the entrenched establishment. As stated in an article in *U.S. News and World Report,* "Geologists and Lawyers Need Not Apply," July 27, 1987, a key question faces education today: "Should adults with first-class education but no pedagogical training be able to teach in the public schools?"

There is formidable resistance to the idea from educational professionals, who have stacked the system against outsiders. Not every school system wants an idealistic newcomer in its midst. Professional jealousy may cause many systems to exclude these retrained scientists.

The answer to the third question, whether parents are ready for an emphasis on academic rigor, will be apparent over time. There is on all sides a call for a return to excellence in this country. And it is widely acknowledged that our economic competitiveness in an information age will rest on an educational foundation. Whether we are ready to translate these general platitudes into individual attitudes will depend on the citizens whose children attend the schools. Wisdom cannot be bought with a bond issue, and knowledge is not acquired by a magical osmosis from the teacher to the pupil. Learning takes time and concentration and hard work on both sides.

Although an inspired teacher can act as a catalytic agent, the act of learning is personal.

Teaching, too, is a personal endeavor, yet the dreams of these would-be teachers are not dreams of personal success. Rather, they dream of contributing, of making a difference by changing the minds of the young. Theirs are dreams of maturity tempered by reality. The successful teachers will be those who approach their work with this vision of changing their world for the better. In its essence, success in life consists in making a difference for good. The challenge of the laid-off employees in the ENCORE class is to make this difference.

Those who land on a teaching trampoline will have an enthusiasm, a tenacity, and a toughness that will enable them to turn the forces of rejection into new energy. They will persevere because they know they are needed. What is the motivation which produces such a phoenix? We believe it is a sense of personal responsibility. It is the wish to give something back to a country that has made much possible for each.

The successful teachers will be those who personalize their quest, those who serve the future of America through serving its young. Great teaching is hard work. Engaging the minds of the active young requires high-energy living. Those who come home at the end of a day of teaching drained of physical energy but filled with psychic energy and enthusiasm for another day are the ones who will make mathematics and science come alive in their classrooms.

Are executives ready for public school education? Is American society ready for excellence? Is there life after lay-off? The answers to all three questions must be affirmative.

CHAPTER 11
CHOOSE YOUR TASK

"He is well paid that is well satisfied." Shakespeare

There is no shortage of needs in our country. We need good schools, improved government, efficient public transportation systems, new ways to care for the indigent. We need to preserve our wildlife, our ozone layer, our natural parks, and our liberties. It is to be hoped that we can alleviate suffering, increase our scientific knowledge, encourage the golden rule and the brotherhood of man. Even the simple and illusive qualities of tenderness and mercy seem sometimes in short supply, superseded by individualism and opportunism.

Whether your passion is the preservation of wildflowers or the improvement of the financial structure of developing nations, there exists a need to fit your hand. Your task will be to make a good match. You will want to match your talents to your cause. No one would be so foolish as to begin a new business without analyzing the match between his personal talents and those required for success in the particular enterprise under consideration. But not enough of us bring this same astute analysis to the choice of volunteer activities. Yet the same rules hold: you will not be a success and your cause will not flourish if there is a mismatch between your talents and your work. It is critically important that you enjoy what you do in your volunteer activities. Absent the payment of money, the knowledge of a job well done and the joy of having done it constitute your full payment for your efforts. In this instance, if you have no aptitude for the task, you have effectively shortchanged yourself.

It is a waste of your time and talents to place yourself in the service of a project for which you have little talent. On the other hand, the happiness which comes from helping others to your fullest ability must surely be one of life's real joys. Your freedom years can open the door to this happiness. Picking your cause is the equivalent to selecting the right key for the door.

One of the urgent causes in our country is the education of our young. Education may be too important to be left to the educators. The many thoughtful citizens who are searching for ways to improve the instruction of our children are in need of help. We interviewed a woman who has dedicated the rest of her life toward this search for excellence in education. She is a busy woman.

Barbara realizes that she has lived a life of good fortune, a life blessed by love and prosperity. She is resolved to repay the privileges she has enjoyed through work designed for the common good. Specifically, she plans to work toward nothing less than a new educational system in this country. Barbara has long way to go, but she has a long range plan to get there, and she expects to live a long time.

In her first stage she will focus on her city, then on her state, and, finally, on the country as a whole. In each stage she will need the talents, the intelligence, and whole-hearted cooperation of thinking and voting citizens. She has every intention of working until she gets it.

Barbara believes in excellence, she believes in education, and she believes rigor is rewarded by joy. Now a widow, Barbara was for thirty-one years married to an astute and affluent banker. Graduates of prestigious East Coast universities, they lived the good life together. Barbara is fifty six now, a slender gentlewoman on the September side of middle age. Five feet two, with eyes of piercing blue, her aristocratic features tanned by the Eastern shore sun, she is a remarkable woman. Our interview was conducted in Washington, D.C., a city which she knows well, and she drove us on a tour of Georgetown as we talked. Her pride in her home, the Maryland shore country, and her pleasure in the centuries-old architecture of the sea coast were evident in her extensive knowledge of the beauties of Georgetown.

As she guided her car expertly through the heavy traffic, she sketched for us the joys and obstacles of trying to do it all: rearing the children, managing the households, helping her husband, squeezing in her own career and ambitions as they seemed to fit best around the careers and ambitions of her husband and her children. When her children were grown and successfully launched in the world, she had gone to law school and earned a law degree. There she was dubiously distinguished by having been the oldest graduate to have been awarded such a degree. Now that she is alone, she has transferred her energies and attention and her astutely focused intelligence on what she considers to be the major problem of this country.

Barbara is convinced that at a time when educators are spending precious time and money in a public search for excellence, they are overlooking a useful model which is very close to hand. She believes that this country needs an academic system modeled on our athletic system. As she puts it, "We need to recognize our academically talented, reward accomplishment, and foster an atmosphere of friendly but serious competition among our children. Giftedness is in short supply, a scarce commodity, and we ought in all instances to promote and enhance the development of our uniquely talented. But we do not. If we are to judge by the evidence in our present school systems, when we educate our young, we honor the physically superior, restrain the mentally superior, and ignore the artistically superior."

By and large she believes, "We do a superior job of encouraging those young people who are athletically gifted, while teaching the others toward mediocrity. Yet each trait is distributed with about the same frequency, and each adds a special dimension to our culture. If we were to treat all our gifted children with the same interest and rewards that we show to our athletically gifted, we could in one generation substantially improve our culture." "For example," she said, "Consider how we treat young boys. If a boy shows superior athletic ability in the fifth or sixth grade he will be singled out for encouragement. Soon he will be put in competition with like students. He will be urged to practice, and he will be coached by a man who was himself a good athlete. By the time he is in high school, his talents will be polished to a fine edge. From childhood on, this boy is apt to be cheered, admired, coached, and nurtured toward excellence.

"But suppose this boy had not been good at basketball, but at mathematics. If his tests reveal that he has exceptional ability in mathematics and logic, one of the first things he is likely to do is to learn to conceal this talent. This particular skill will not bring him the admiration of his classmates. Nor is his school likely to have a fifth-grade teacher who is capable of coaching him in number theory and analysis. He learns to conceal this talent behind a mask of indifference. Soon the mask becomes real, and his performance is aimed toward the norm, the mediocre. We are an elitist nation when it comes to athletics. We are egalitarian when it comes to academics."

Barbara believes that change will require massive restructuring. Patchwork won't do it. Beginning in her city, she has enlisted the aid of others to design nothing less than a new philosophy and a new system of education, one in which mediocrity is replaced by excellence, one to which each thinking adult is dedicated. She is working to design a financial and legal structure to support this change. She truly believes that beauty is truth, and truth beauty. Running through her conversation is the conviction that a life lived in the zestful search for excellence is a life of happiness.

The sun was setting when she drove us back to our hotel. Paused at a traffic light, waiting to make a left turn, she summed up her entire philosophy as we slowed our talk to look at the faces of the pedestrians crossing in front of her car. Most were well dressed, post-middle aged people, appearing tired and glum as they hastened across the street, their thoughts focused elsewhere. Gently and purposefully Barbara eased her car toward them, then urgently beamed her philosophy in their direction. "Smile," she said,

"Smile! and pay attention to where you are going!"

Sometimes a hobby can evolve into a cause, as did Lady Bird Johnson's devotion to the wildflower boom. The National Wildflower Research Center is an outgrowth of the former first lady's love of the wildflowers and pine thickets of her Texas girlhood. In 1952, Mrs. Johnson invited others to join her in establishing the National Wildlife Research Center to encourage people to preserve and use these lovely plants in landscaping with native species. As quoted in a *Smithsonian* article, she stated, "I had the notion that in this way I might give back something to the country I've loved—pay my rent, so to speak, for the space I've taken up and the good times I've had." The beauty of the flowers obscures their practicality. The crimson of acres of Indian Paintbrush growing by miles of freeways provides low-maintenance erosion protection; the azure of Texas Bluebonnets changes monotony into beauty. Wildflowers stabilize the soil, save millions of dollars per year in highway maintenance, and provide lovely reminders of the balance that can be achieved between beauty and utility. Lady Bird's hobby has become a popular cause.

Most of us have more than one cause about which we care deeply. Generally, our task is not to find a cause to champion, but rather to select from among the many those few to which we will give our time and talents. Your answers to the following questions will serve as a barometer to help you choose:
1. How much do I know about the problem?
2. How important do others consider this task to be?
3. How much do I care about the outcome?
4. How much time am I willing to give to it?

5. What is the match between my talents and those needed for success?
6. Will I enjoy the work?
7. Will I feel satisfaction from success in it?

Now is the time for passion. Whatever you decide to do, do it with all your heart. When you pick a cause, let it be one that truly matters to you. This is not the time for modest aims nor timid hopes. Aim for an outcome that you believe to be truly important.

At a recent conference at the Ohio State University, the amazing Grace Hopper, retired Rear Admiral of the U.S. Navy, urged a capacity crowd toward no less a goal than true leadership. She has earned the right to do it. Grace Hopper led the way toward the information age. She served her country as a naval officer and programmer for the first large-scale computer in the land, the Mark I. Now a legend in her own time, at the age of 81 she still dazzles her listeners as she urges younger generations toward clear thinking and positive leadership. She has lived her speech. Physically frail and tiny, she is an intellectual giant. Her message is potent: "You manage things—you lead people!"

Whether your mission is to speak to capacity crowds at major universities or to work quietly in your own home town on a task that badly needs doing, let your cause be one you believe in. When you give the time and talents of your freedom years you are giving a gift beyond price, one that will enrich both you and your world.

Do not hesitate to let your reach exceed your grasp. Not all of Grace Hopper's audience will become true leaders, but some will, and their work will enrich the nation. Your own cause may be just as important. You may affect the future of many.

We live in a time when change is coming fast. You can influence change in your world. Whether you choose to concentrate your efforts on your neighborhood or to design a strategy to influence the nation, what you do can make a difference. Choose a task you can commit to. Choose a task you can love.

CHAPTER 12
EXPAND YOUR HORIZONS

"A man's reach should exceed his grasp, or what's a heaven for?" Browning

For each of us there comes a time when we are required to examine the fabric of our lives. This moment comes early for the fortunate few, and thereafter their decisions are informed by the knowledge of who they are and what they wish to become. To know who we are and to set our course on the basis of this knowledge is to have an internal radar that continually guides us along the path toward becoming our best.

Many drift through young adulthood and even into middle age without this critical knowledge. Without that inner knowledge we drift at the mercy of random forces. It is this targeted radar that distinguishes the salmon from the carp: the salmon that swims against the current in order to fulfill his destiny is universally admired; the carp, lazily drifting to his bloated old age, has become a symbol for idleness.

This is a chapter about salmon, about continued energy and expanded horizons. We shall not spend time on the carp. In a very real sense it is a chapter about happiness, especially a form of happiness earned through service to others.

If you have been one whose internal radar has guided you toward success you have already experienced its rewards, and retirement is not the time to stop. It is simply the time to refocus your talents. Nor is it always necessary to create a new project in order to give scope to these talents. More often, the projects are already in place, initiated by others of similar views, ready and worthy of your best efforts and energy. Many have found expanded horizons through personal service in hospitals and schools and social agencies. Others have turned a special talent into a vocation.

If your career has been that of an executive, you may qualify for one of our country's special organizations of retirees. Its advertisements state, "We are looking for retired managers to work hard in a strange place with no pay." The advertisement refers to monetary pay. There is no limit to the earnings in enjoyment, satisfaction, new experiences, and new friends. But the requirements are stringent. Applicants must be willing to work with their heads, their hands, and their hearts.

This special organization is the International Executives Service Corps. Founded by David Rockefeller during the Lyndon Johnson administration, and flourishing still, it enjoys the blessings of the government while remaining a private enterprise supported by private funding. Its basic purpose is to help others help themselves.

Its disparagers called it the paunch corps, or, worse, the fat man's Peace Corps. But *Fortune* magazine wrote that, "For all the jibes at haunch, paunch, and jowl, the Executive Peace Corps is performing wonders for struggling foreign businesses." The reason is simple. It is surprising how much a man or woman can accomplish if he or she does not worry about who gets the credit.

The retired executive who is chosen to serve in this special group will find the job to be part ambassador for America, part business coach and advocate of good management, and full time servant leader. The aim of each enterprise—and there have now been more than 10,000 successful enterprises in 84 different countries—is to shore up freedom in developing nations by promoting the sound management of private enterprise. This is done through the transfer of knowledge, both of technology and management. Applicants are expected to be shirt-sleeve ambassadors and hands-on experts. Arm chair experts need not apply.

The qualifications of this overseas ambassador who will serve in the IESC have been defined over time.

1. He/she is a manager of proved capacity.
2. He/she is a person who has done well in the United States.
3. He/she is active.
4. He/she is mature and modest.
5. He/she is carefully selected.

The compensation system has been clearly defined, also. Volunteers give their time and know-how, receiving travel and living expenses for themselves and spouse. The term per project is usually three months. The dimensions of service to clients are sometimes extended through the practice of Piggyback and Diagnostic concepts. This practice may make the volunteers' expertise available to a second client in the general geographic area, thus saving recruiting time and transatlantic air fare.

Whether the assignment is to a shoe factory in Turkey, a plastics plant in Ghana, an automotive supplier in Brazil, or a hotel in Haiti, the executive on loan must be able to combine know-how with do-how. Academic expertise alone is insufficient. The man or woman who represents IESC must be able to show as well as tell. If the job calls for it, he or she must be able to wade in the rice paddies or sew in the shoe factory.

The project which in 1986 marked the 10,000th successful enterprise serves as a case in point. The IESC answered a client's call for help in an agribusiness project in Ecuador. The problem was to improve milk production on a milk cattle ranch. The expert sent to assist the ranch was himself a ranch owner, and the problem was solved in three months.

Most projects are measured in months, and success is expected to be measurable in terms of the balance sheet. The IESC is a group with the underlying motto that it is good business to do good. Founded on the premise that free enterprise is an exportable product, its ambassadors have found an extraordinary joy in their work.

David Rockefeller's dream has been made a reality almost entirely by retirees, men and women who have retired from successful careers. Their flexibility, innovation and adaptability have dispelled the myths which equate age with stoginess. The challenges and hardships which are the built-in components of developing nations are overcome with style.

The workers in this corps have been building bridges between worlds. As ambassadors of the free market economy they have made friends for America in ways that transcend the barriers of language. They have managed to link the common goals of humanity.

Like the Marine Corps, IESC is always looking for a few good men and women. If you believe you can contribute, write to International Executive Service Corps, 622 Third Avenue, New York, NY 10017.

The path to suigeneris need not take you out of the country, and you need not have been an executive to qualify.

When projects require specific talents it sometimes happens that an individual is literally drafted into service. When this happened to George he entered the busiest phase of his life.

In 1977 George was the Assistant to the President of a large employee-owned newspaper. A long-term employee, he had begun as a reporter, had served as managing editor, and was a member of the board of directors when the paper was sold by the employees to a large East Coast firm. George knows the inner workings of his city as well as he knows the inner workings of his newspaper, a synergistic combination with value immediately apparent to the incoming chief executive. When the new C.E.O. took over, George became his assistant, operating as his ambassador within the community.

This new career turn has brought George more fun than he would have guessed a man in his seventies could have. Active on many boards, he advises the publisher on the distribution of funds of the newspaper's philanthropic foundation, and serves on the Downtown Council. He is on the board of one of the nation's most prestigious foundations, effectively assessing the needs of the community and faithfully translating these needs to the publisher. In all of his service, George's career aim is to help his newspaper effectively serve its constituency. Although George performs as an ambassador, his is not a political job, for a newspaper informs rather than directs. George's rare and valuable combination of intelligence, experience, and instinct is enhanced by his age.

George does not regard himself as a tenured employee. He serves at the pleasure of his C.E.O., a time-honored condition of ambassadorial duties. Not unlike another venerable institution, service is his most important product.

Service and suigeneris are often concurrent, and Bill Jones is building his path to suigeneris with his own hands. Bill's usual work week is 50 to 60 hours. He may be the highest paid worker in Magazine, Arkansas, for he is being paid in a rare coin—the coin of true enjoyment. The week we interviewed him was typical: On Monday and Tuesday, he worked on a four-man team, painting the wood trim on the sturdy brick church that is the hallmark of his little town. The team reported for work early Monday morning and finished the job at 4:30 p.m. the next day.

Wednesday, Bill plowed and hoed his garden, almost an acre of ground. Soon he will plant enough corn, potatoes, purple hull peas, improved pinto beans and green beans to feed a multitude. Bill's wife, Doris, will spend the summer canning and freezing, cooking or giving away the beautiful bounty from this vegetable garden. On Thursday Bill repeated the operations of Wednesday, an effort identical except for location. This time he put in a garden for an eighty year old neighbor, a widow whose forty-three year old retarded son requires most of her time and efforts.

Bill and Doris gave themselves a small vacation on

Friday and Saturday, traveling to Tulsa, Oklahoma, to attend the festive wedding of the son of a boyhood friend. But they got up early at 5 a.m. on Sunday to drive back to Magazine in time for church and Bill's responsibilities as a church trustee and member of the finance committee. Bill is not one to talk much about his religion, probably because he is too busy living it.

During his 34 years as an equipment specialist with the United States Army Missile Command, Bill became a maintenance expert, a man with responsibilities for the maintenance of army missile depots around the world. After decades of working with his head, he rejoices in the opportunity to work with this hands and his heart. When he and Doris moved back to her home town, where scenic Mount Magazine rises beyond their back door, they felt the best part of their life was just beginning. Bill figures there are lots of people willing to tell others what to do. As for himself, Bill prefers to practice rather than preach.

The months of February and March were landmark times for Magazine, because the townspeople reestablished and improved their fire department. Bill was in the middle of the project. Not only does he serve on the City Council of Magazine and the Magazine Improvement Club, organizations that successfully obtained a federal grant for new fire engines and materials to build new bays to house them, but he was a worker on the team which rebuilt and expanded the fire department building. The entire 34 ft. by 25 ft. building was built by volunteer labor. Bill did a little bit of everything. He poured footings, mixed cement, carried concrete blocks, welded, raised rafters and poured floors. For the total team, it was a labor of love.

Bill has never been happier. While he applauds those who looked for new worlds to conquer, he and Doris have found the good life right in their own back yard.

CHAPTER 13
PERSUADE OTHERS

"So long as we love we serve." Robert Louis Stevenson

The process of persuasion is the keystone upon which our civilization rests. Persuasion is the basis of our orderly system of living. The discovery of the wheel and the development of the arts of persuasion both have their roots in man's dim past. Most of us long ago concluded that we are not likely to be called on to re-invent the wheel. Some of us, however, may need a refresher course in the arts and science of persuasion.

The sophistication of persuasion enabled man to move beyond carrying a club to get what he wanted. When brute force was the only method of satisfying needs and wants, life was simply a struggle for survival, a struggle won by the swift and the strong. We have progressed considerably from the days of the cave man. But those of us who have spent our careers in the corporate world may still carry a mental club and depend on the principle known as the "survival of the fittest." Whether we were accustomed to being on the giving end or the receiving end—the clouter or the cloutee—we remember the effects of clout.

When you retire it is time to put the concept of clout into permanent storage. Clout is to the retiree what the club is to civilization. The society to which you are moving has its wheels oiled, not by clout, but by the powers of persuasion.

The retiree who moves from the status of Very Important Person to that of a Formerly Important Person, from V.I.P. to F.I.P., will achieve success only to the extent to which he or she can adjust to this new reality.

We recently attended the divestiture of a V.I.P. This man was a banker who was retired with the usual banquet, parties and publicity used to ease out a high official to make room for the eager young tigers crouching for the spring. This V.I.P., however, was somehow unaware that he had inadvertently become an F.I.P.

The F.I.P. received his first disenchantment sometime later, when his usual table at the club somehow was not reserved for him with the same sanctity as before. Somehow, his jokes were not as funny, his wife was not as popular, and their social calendar was not as crowded. Finally he was forced to accept the fact that all through the years he had occupied the position as V.I.P. he had never really been important—only his job had been important. His title had carried the clout, and he had been in the position to do favors and advance the interests of others. His importance had permitted him to promote and elevate. Absent the ability to materially affect the lives of others in a business situation, his importance faded with his favors. It is sad to see a man who honestly believes his future is behind him. Often at this point the F.I.P. is tempted to begin to improve those around him rather than improving his own life.

We later saw the F.I.P. at the grocery store pushing his wife's shopping cart. He was at that time engaged in giving his wife's purchasing habits his careful scrutiny and undivided attention, while considerably improving them in the process. If he were to have listened carefully to his soliloquy on the inordinately high cost of a pint of strawberries and his wife's unmitigated extravagance in the purchase of the same, he might have begun to understand his true message. It went something like this: "acknowledge my financial expertise; give me the respect which my subordinates used to give me; reassure me that I am still a V.I.P."

The solution to our F.I.P.'s problem is not to be found in the improvement of the shopping habits of his spouse. She is apt to be afflicted with incipient insubordination about this time, anyway. Rather, the solution lies in reality therapy, in recognizing the need for new living patterns in a new stage of life.

Reality is a harsh law, but if we recognize it and accept it, we can avoid surprise and needless suffering. The same emotional maturity which allows its acceptance will bring with it a real sense of relief. To substitute skillful persuasion for undisguised clout is to step into an advanced state of civilization.

Those who advance in the state of retirement are those who have learned the art of persuading others—the art of selling ideas to others. The power of persuading other people is the essence of our existence. It is the balance wheel that gives stability to our economic system, harmony to our social system, and serenity to life itself.

Our ability to influence others affects our lives to an enormous extent, probably more than any other single quality we possess. Yet too few have given this matter sufficient study or consideration. The decades of your future will offer you ample opportunity for practice. Whether your powers of persuasion are well-polished, underdeveloped, or in need of remediation, there can be no better time to consider their importance. Regardless of how you spend your time, you will deal with people the rest of your life. And in most of these dealings you will be called on to persuade, to convince, and to sell your ideas. There is a three-step formula which can open the door of opportunity for you.

Step number one: Be sure you are understood. This simple and basic step is the one most often overlooked. Yet lawyers agree that more than half the controversies that arise among people are caused, not by differences of opinion or even ability to agree, but rather by lack of understanding. There is misunderstanding even about the simple process of making ourselves understood.

Are you articulate? Do you make your thoughts clear to others? Don't be too sure. If you will take the time to listen to a play back on a tape recorder of the next meeting you attend or the next presentation you make, you may be surprised at what you hear. Even though you may have been full of your subject and completely informed on your topic, it is possible that your audience may have missed your message. If you assume your audience to be as well informed as you are you may create blind spots of understanding.

People are not persuaded by what we say, but rather by what they understand. Those who try to impress often confuse. There is greatness in simplicity, and brilliance in brevity.

The Lord's prayer consists of fifty-seven words, none more than two syllables. The Declaration of Independence, which revolutionized the New World, can be read by a school child in five minutes. Lincoln's Gettysburg Address is splendidly simple. Words are the fingers that mold the mind of man. And the mind of another is much more pliable when your own approach is direct. A confused mind hardens like cement, and often much faster.

We can say almost the same thing in two different ways and get two entirely different reactions. When a gentleman tells a lady, "You are truly a vision," she usually smiles and feels complimented. If he says, "You really are a sight," he is headed for trouble. When he says, "When I look into your eyes, all time stands still," he has usually attained her full attention. Yet, if he were to say, "Your face would stop a clock," he is on dangerous ground. Although words are the fingers that mold the mind, they still must be the right words, and easily understood. The first requirement of the art of persuasion is that for your listeners to understand you, you must make your meaning clear.

Step Number Two: You must truly believe in what you are saying. In order for others to think, believe, and act as you desire, you must first think, believe, and act upon it yourself. We cannot give what we do not have. We cannot be convincing until we ourselves are convinced. We cannot persuade others to enthusiasm until we ourselves are full of enthusiasm.

Enthusiasm is contagious. It spreads faster than a disease, because enthusiasm is controlled excitement. Its origin is in the Greek word "Theus,", which means "the God within us." Your happiness in your retirement years will be directly proportional to the enthusiasm which you bring to your days.

There is a statue in England which is actually a

monument to enthusiasm. It tells the story of how the game of Rugby began. Rugby is an offspring of soccer, and began with a spontaneous event.

The statue is one of an excited boy leaning down and picking up a ball. At the base of the statue is the inscription: *With a fine disregard for the rules, he picked up the ball and ran.*

The statue and inscription tell a true story. An important game of soccer was taking place between two English schools. A boy more gifted with enthusiasm and school spirit than with experience was sent into the game during the closing minutes. Forgetting all the rules, including the rule that a soccer player does not touch the ball with his hands, and conscious only that the ball had to be at the goal line within seconds if his school were to be victorious, the boy picked up the ball in his arms and started the sprint of his life to the goal line.

The confused officials and players were frozen in disbelief. But the spectators went wild at the boy's uncontrollable excitement and school spirit, and they stood up and cheered one ringing cheer after another. This memorable day marked the birth of a new national sport. The new game was named Rugby in honor of the school where it happened.

This story is an example of the power of enthusiasm and spirit. Armed with practically nothing else, many an individual has accomplished wonders. To believe deeply in a cause and to become excited over its merits is truly a valuable asset. To possess this wonderful quality we must first be devoid of suspicion. We must remove the cloak of cynicism, and concentrate on playing the game. The game of life is ready to be played when you are.

Step Number Three: Finally, we approach the third

quality necessary to complete the formula of persuasion: Be of service to others. If you are attempting to persuade me toward any action or belief, please tell me what it will do for me—how it will serve my interest. For me to be persuaded, I need to believe you are bringing me a benefit or serving my interests. Unless you can show me some advantage I am missing or some benefit I can enjoy, then regardless of your enthusiasm I shall remain unconvinced.

We cannot prosper except by bringing prosperity to others. We cannot become rich except through enriching others.

Cavett once had the privilege of meeting the great poet, Edwin Markham, and he asked, "Mr. Markham, which of your poems is your favorite?" He expected the poet to mention "Lincoln," or "The Man with the Hoe." Mr. Markham stood, threw his head back, and said, "I wrote four lines which I treasure more than all else." And looking up he recited:

"He drew a circle and shut me out,
Heretic, rebel, a thing to flout,
But love and I had the wit to win,
We drew a circle and took him in."

This poem illustrates one of the great lessons of persuasion. In order to convince a person we are not required to pierce the circle he draws around himself, or to break down the wall of protection he builds. If we truly have the spirit of service, if our concern is truly the other person's interest, we have but to draw a larger circle.

If our motives are honorable, if our prime concern is to perform some service for another or for the larger community, resistance fades away and is replaced by our dominant concern for the welfare of others. Many emotions can be faked, but sincere interest in helping others is not one of them. Unless the compulsion for service exceeds our passion for gain—unless the dollar we earn is only a by-product of the service we render—there will not be enough of those dollars to make a difference anyway.

Cavett likes to say that if the prime consideration in any effort is simply to make money, dollars will slip through your fingers like a handful of water. But if your major concern is to solve another's problem, pretty soon dollars are apt to come around and beg to play in your back yard just to see what kind of person you are.

Cavett's favorite story is a French fable that illustrates the human need to be of service, a fable entitled "The Servant of the Kingdom":

The king's cupbearer was walking in a dense forest near the palace one day. He was approached by a giant genie who said, "You have been a good man, and I will grant you one wish, but be careful what you ask for. I will grant you only one."

The man thought for a while and said, "All my life I have served others. In fact, my title is, 'Servant of the Kingdom'. For the rest of my life I would like for people to wait on me and serve me. I want the tables turned. In the future I want people to do for me."

The genie said, "Are you sure this is what you really want? My power is limited. I can grant only one wish."

"Yes, yes," was the cupbearer's eager reply.

Sure enough, when the man went back to the castle a footman opened the door for him. When he tried to serve the king, someone else had taken his place. Servants dressed him, fed him, and waited on him. Regardless of how hard he tried, he could do nothing for anyone, and everything was done for him.

The first month was fabulous. The second month it became irritating. Finally, during the third month it became unbearable.

So the man headed for the forest to search for the genie, and finally found him. Humbly he said to the genie, "I've decided that having people wait on me isn't as much pleasure as I thought. I'd like to return to my old job. I want to be the Servant of the Kingdom again and wait on other people."

The genie said, "I'm sorry but I cannot help you. I told you at the time that I could grant only one wish."

But the man said, "You don't understand. I want to serve other people. It is far more rewarding to give than to receive. I don't want others to wait on me."

Again the genie explained, shaking his head, "I am without the power to help you."

In desperation the man begged, "But you must help me—You MUST! Please let me do for others. I'd rather be in hell than not be able to serve my fellow man!"

The genie, as he vanished, said sorrowfully, "My friend, where do you think you have been for the last ninety days?"

CHAPTER 14
LIVE HARMONIOUSLY WITH OTHERS

"The heart has reasons the mind never heard of!" Cavett Robert

A wealth of self-help books can be found to assist us toward achieving harmony with others. All begin with the same principle. In order to live harmoniously with others, you must first get in harmony with yourself. As one noted speaker in the field explains it, you must first get your own instrument in tune. In this chapter, we are going to discuss ways of tuning your inner self, and then follow this by learning to harmonize with the differences of others.

Rule Number One: To get in harmony with yourself, concentrate first on becoming acquainted with yourself. Be truthful with yourself. Stop comparing yourself with all those other people with whom you have spent your life. Stop sitting in judgment on yourself, and take the time to find out who you are, what it takes to make you happy, and what you really want out of life. Your happiness chart will yield much information if you will keep it faithfully and well. If you will be as fair with yourself as you would be with others, you will find that an honest look at the happy parts of your life will tell you volumes.

Forget about the "oughts" and the "shoulds." If ever in your life you are going to understand your inner self, it is now in this freedom phase of your existence. Try to be kind and decent to yourself, as kind as you would be to anyone you love. Face the fact that you are not angelic, not infallible, and not omnipotent. But you are unique, a creature of the personality and character which you yourself have created, and a person of inestimable worth. None of us is perfect, yet each can seek and find the road to suigeneris and revel in the journey.

Now is the time to take stock of your life so far. If you have not yet lived a life which is true to your best self, this is not the time for despair, but for rejoicing in your gift of another chance. Your future gives you the opportunity to discard those habits and attitudes which are not in harmony with your real self. Do you know any one who is perfect? Do you know many who are not? Permit yourself to share the characteristics of the human race. Retirement can provide the opportunity to acknowledge the essence of humanity—that the persons we have become are all intriguingly flawed, inordinately precious, and joyously individual. For better or for worse, you are who you are.

In your search for your true self, learn how to be alone with yourself. Learn to welcome solitude as the friend it can be. The person who shadows his friends a bit too closely, who keeps tabs on the actions of all his adult children as though they all required the careful guidance of childhood, even the person who supervises his wife in her housekeeping, is suffering from the fear of solitude. The F.I.P. we met in the grocery store, helping his wife toward improvement, would be happier if he concentrated first on learning to live with himself. It is idle to try to improve others before we have finished the task of improving ourselves.

Louise recalls with chagrin a scene from her young womanhood when she became vividly aware of this principle. As a young matron with her first child, she was just beginning to assume her community responsibilities, and was rather self importantly enjoying her role as a church worker and community activist. In this stage of her life she returned to Arkansas for a visit with her parents, who had spent their lives responsibly loving the people who were their neighbors. From her newly-acquired sense of responsibility, Louise said to her mother, "Mama, do you sometimes worry because Daddy has not ever formally joined the church?" Without disturbing the rhythm of her rocking chair, her mother replied, "Louise, when you have become as good a woman as your father is a man, you come back home and we will worry together about your father's church membership!"

Rule Number Two: Learn to enjoy other people for their uniqueness. Extend the same privilege to your friends and acquaintances as you are now extending to yourself. Permit your friends and relatives to be unique. When you stop categorizing people according to race, or age, or social class, or bank account, or occupation, you will find your world to be much broader and your life to be more pleasurable. By paying attention to the special talents and quirks of others you will have the opportunity to fill some blank spaces in the canvas which is the picture of your own life. When you take the time to understand the interests and attitudes of your friends you will have expanded your own frame of reference. Try not to regard yourself as a lonely little petunia in an onion patch, but rather as a durable daisy in a perennial garden.

Dr. Joseph C. Robert, former president of Hampden Sydney College, tells of the suburban householder whose entire yard was covered with dandelions. Reacting with the conventional wisdom, he hated the dandelions. Obtaining all the advice he could get, he tried every method he could think of to get rid of them. He grubbed and he sprayed and he cut and he complained, but, still, up came the dandelions. Finally he wrote a letter to that last refuge of all citizens... The Government. In a letter to the United States Department of Agriculture he narrated in detail his fruitless efforts... mechanical, biological, and chemical. Finally came the solution from Washington, "There is only one thing left to do. You must learn to love dandelions!"

When you have learned to love the differences of others and even to harmonize with these differences, life gets infinitely easier. We can, in fact, welcome these differences and use them. Differences in viewpoints lead to objections from others, and every successful attempt at harmony is based on the principle of harmonizing with objections. This fact is the basis for our next rule.

Rule Number Three: Learn to harmonize with the objections of others. This principle is not confined to commercial selling, but applies to every phase of our lives. Unless it is applied to family life, business life, social life and community activities, it would not be a sound and consistent principle. Truth is the whole. To fragment our behavior into one set of principles for personal living and another for community life is an error. Objections are useful for they furnish unmistakable clues as to the thinking of others. Without them we are helpless. In order to live harmoniously with others, we first must know the basis of our differences and this basis is evidenced by objections.

Beware of the person who will not give any clue as to what he is thinking, the person who will never furnish you with any objection from which to measure your position. The person who is reluctant to give another a glimpse of his thoughts or feelings is a lonely person, insecure and vaguely afraid. These are the people who are afraid of losing something of themselves if they share with others... even sharing an opinion becomes an anticipated loss. Avoid becoming such a person, and avoid the temptation to be less than sympathetic with the objections of others. Sincerely expressed differences are clues to individuality.

In order to learn the proper manner of dealing with an objection we must first know why a person is objecting. We cannot suggest a remedy for anything unless we first know what is causing the ailment. Psychologists tell us it is futile to treat a result. The only effective manner of helping a situation is to treat the cause. So it is obvious that the first step in harmonizing with objections is to probe into the background and find out just what causes the person to think and feel the way he does.

If you were sick and went to a doctor's office the doctor would first conduct an examination. He would take your temperature, feel your pulse, put you through a series of diagnostic tests, and ask you a series of probing questions. He would search for the cause, the reason behind your symptoms. After this examination he would make his analysis and prescribe treatment, a course of action directed at the cause behind your sickness. This is the professional approach, and it instills confidence that the treatment will deal with the cause and result in a cure.

If, however, the same doctor had seemed unconcerned with your symptoms, had neglected to examine you or to subject you to any scientific tests, but had immediately begun to discuss his treatment with you, you would be right to feel apprehension. If he concentrated on the cure while ignoring the cause, you would probably begin to suspect him of indifference...even quackery. And you would most likely be correct.

But how many people today are trying to correct situations and symptoms in daily living and are failing miserably because they refuse to acknowledge the source or to eradicate the cause? Cavett says that sin is similar to a toothache. Each has to become almost unbearable before we are willing to remove the cause.

When Lady Macbeth was suffering the anguish of a guilty conscience, in desperation she pleaded with the court physician:

"Can't thou not minister to a mind diseased;
Pluck from the memory a rooted sorrow;
Raze out the written troubles of the brain;
And with some sweet oblivious antidote
Cleanse the stuff'd bosom of that perilous stuff
Which weights upon the heart?"

The reply which Shakespeare gave through the physician is one of the classics of all literature:

"Therein the patient must minister to himself."

Nothing and no one can help change any situation

until the cause is admitted and treated. Why do people object to the suggestions of others? If we know the causes of objections we are in a position to deal with them. Some people object because they are offended. This is an emotional objection, one without logical foundation, and usually hopeless to change. This is fortunately, a situation which applies to only a small proportion of the population.

Many people object simply because they do not understand a situation. Here, education is the answer. A confused mind automatically says no. Sometimes it is less embarrassing to object on some basis that is not real than it is to admit that one does not understand the situation. Never assume that those who object to your ideas have a full understanding of your proposition. Think ahead of them, but talk behind them. Constantly ask if you are making yourself clear.

One of the main reasons people object is that they are actually afraid to make decisions. Most people are not accustomed to making major decisions. Did you ever sit and watch people in a restaurant trying to decide what they will order from the menu? Ninety-five percent of people are imitators and five percent are originators, primarily because most people dislike making decisions—or do not know how to. If ever in your life you are going to make your own decisions, the time is now. Take charge of yourself. You will be amazed at how rewarding it will be.

Sometimes a person's objection is really only a question. Actually, he is interested and only searching for knowledge. Even people who really want a product or service or who are attracted to an idea often object because they want to delay making a decision. Every objection except the first kind, those which spring from being offended, can be used to advantage as a guide to the person's thinking, provided we realize what is back of each objection. The following guidelines are useful as pointing to pitfalls to avoid:

Don't be too quick to decide what the other person's real objection is, and, even more important, what is behind it. Hear him out completely. Then repeat the objection, and ask him if you understood him correctly. Of the several steps that should be taken to solve a problem, by far the most important is to determine at the beginning the exact nature of the problem. Don't jump to conclusions. Ascertain accurately and fully the real problem in the other's mind.

Do not interrupt the other person when he is voicing an objection. Do not dignify an objection by putting undue importance upon it. On the other hand, never ridicule an objection. The magic formula for dealing effectively with objections voiced by another can be divided into four steps. When you receive an objection (1) act delighted, (2) treat it as a question, (3) get the commitment that this is the only question, and (4) finally use the same reasoning which the person gave for objecting as his reason for agreeing.

This sounds simple, it is simple, and it works. It is very easy for a person experienced in the art of persuasion to act delighted about an objection because actually he is delighted. To have an objection received enthusiastically is most disarming, and lays the perfect foundation for the other three steps.

Recently a client of Cavett's bought a motel in Mesa, Arizona. Shortly thereafter he brought a letter into Cavett's law office. The letter was from the person who owned a competitive motel next door, a person who was very bitter. His competitor stated that Cavett's client's fence was two feet over on his property. Cavett assured the client that he would represent him, but months went by without any word. Finally, one day, Cavett met his client on the street. He tells the story as follows:

"Cavett," the client said, "I began to wonder if there was not a way to avoid all the commotion and hard feelings of a lawsuit. So I wrote the fellow whose property was next to mine and told him that I didn't blame him a bit. If I were in his shoes I would feel the same way. If the fence is on his property it ought to come down. I asked him, however, why it was necessary to go through all the expense and hard feelings of a lawsuit. We could get a surveyor ourselves and easily find where the property line lies. Furthermore, after we had found out just where the property lies, the two of us could move the fence without hiring anyone else. I told him that would give us a chance to become acquainted as long as we were going to be neighbors."

"Pretty soon," the client continued, "I got a short note in reply to my letter. The fellow told me that the fence was going to remain exactly where it was. He said that there was a doubt in everyone's mind as to just who owned the two feet of property, but that if I would have my lawyer draw up the papers he would sign a quitclaim deed and clear up the dispute."

"The fact is," he said, "I have gotten to know this fellow and we have become friends. We are going to form a partnership and put all the property in our joint names. By doing this we can build four more units in the space that separates the two motels. In the future we will have one office. He and his wife play bridge almost every night with my wife and me, and whoever is dummy can answer the bell. It will save a lot of time that way."

Step Number Four is the logical extension of the first three. Be a friend. When you talk with people, listen. Focus on their words and on their emotions. Really listen, and really care about the message they are sending to you. Practice empathy, involve your thoughts, and your feelings in the situation of those in the world around you. Resolve that each day you will do something thoughtful for others and do it without any expectation of reward other than their happiness. We cannot improve on the formula given by the Master Teacher 2,000 years ago: "Do unto others as you would have them do unto you."

III. THE REWARDS

CHAPTER 15
ENJOY THE LIFE YOU HAVE EARNED

'All animals except man know that the chief business of life is to enjoy it." Samuel Butler

In recent years we have heard a lot about quality time. Actually, quality has little to do with time. You may experience more happiness in one exhilarating moment than in weeks of ordinary existence. For some, the pursuit of happiness is an activity which is the modern equivalent of the ancient quest for the Holy Grail—a treasure perpetually located in the future. Some may know contentment but believe happiness to be elusive.

Contentment itself may be enough. The dictionary defines happiness as joy, a state of well-being or contentment. A young friend of ours uses "joy" as a verb. She says, "I was joyed!" It may help you get a perspective on your own experiences if you ask yourself the question, "When am I joyed?"

The following table was designed to help you analyze when you were joyed, what joyed you, and the extent and the frequency of that enjoyment. Please take the time to fill out your enjoyment chart. It will remind you of what you enjoy and help you measure the proportion of your time which you allocate to activities that make you happy. If this list does not include your favorite activities, write them in the blank spaces at the end.

In order to complete your own satisfaction score, record your enjoyment responses and your frequency responses in the following table. For this computation we will list each response according to its weighted number. Fill out your enjoyment chart by recording these numbers to measure your enjoyment:

Very Much = 3, Moderately = 2, Some = 1, Not at All = −1; On the frequency chart, Daily = 3, Weekly = 2, Sometimes = 1, and Never = −1.

As an illustration of the scoring technique, please go through the following sample computation: Ann's enjoyment scores on the first few items were:

PART I
How Much Do You Enjoy It?

Activity	Very Much +3	Moderately +2	Some +1	Not at All −1
1. Gardening				−1
2. Photography		2		
3. Drawing and Painting			1	
4. Crafts	3			
5. Acting				−1

Ann's frequency scores were:

PART II
Frequency

Activity	Daily +3	Weekly +2	Sometimes +1	Never −1
1. Gardening		2		
2. Photography			1	
3. Drawing and Painting				−1
4. Crafts			1	
5. Acting				−1

Ann's satisfaction scores were:

	Enjoyment Part I	Frequency Part II	Scores Multiply I x II
1. Gardening	−1	2	−2
2. Photography	2	1	2
3. Drawing and Painting	1	−1	−1
4. Crafts	3	1	3
5. Acting	−1	−	1
Sum Total (Ann's Satisfaction Score)			3

Because she disliked gardening, yet did it weekly, her gardening scores multipled as $(-1)(2) = -2$. She actually enjoyed photography, but did not engage in it often; she was mildly interested in drawing and never did it; she enjoyed crafts very much, although she seldom engaged in them. Ann's only consistent pair of scores described her reaction to acting: she had no interest in acting (-1) and never acted (-1); these two negative but consistent responses multiplied to score a positive one.

Ann could considerably increase her satisfaction by eliminating gardening, which she dislikes, and increasing her involvement in photography and with crafts, which she enjoys very much. If she were to do this, her satisfaction in life would improve dramatically, as would her scores:

	Enjoyment	Frequency	Scores
1. Gardening	−1	never (−1)	+1
2. Photography	2	weekly (2)	+4
3. Drawing and Painting	1	never (−1)	−1
4. Crafts	3	daily (3)	9
5. Acting	−1	never (−1)	1
Sum Total (Ann's Satisfaction Score)			+15

TABLE VI: YOUR ENJOYMENT CHART

A
How Much Do You Enjoy This Activity?

Activity	Very Much	Moderately	Some	Not At All
	+3	+2	+1	−1

B
How Often Do You Do This?

Daily	Weekly	Sometimes	Never
+3	+2	+1	−1

Satisfaction Scores
Enjoyment X Frequency

1. Gardening
2. Photography
3. Drawing and Painting
4. Crafts
5. Acting
6. Playing a Musical Instrument
7. Writing
8. Cooking
9. Housework
10. Yard Work
11. Playing Cards or Other Card Games
12. Sewing
13. Driving
14. Public Speaking
15. Singing
16. Tennis
17. Golf
18. Hiking/Walking
19. Dancing
20. Working on Automobiles
21. Television
22. Movies
23. Theater
24. Concerts
25. Museums
26. Spectator Sports
27. Parties (guest)
28. Entertaining
29. Hunting
30. Fishing
31. Shopping
32. Travel
33. Study
34. Skiing
35. Sailing
36. Team Sports
37. Others

Please complete your responses by multiplying your scores for each activity. Algebraic rules: plus times plus = plus; plus times minus = minus; minus times minus = plus. Thus, when you engage often in an activity you enjoy, you compute your score by multiplying a plus by a plus. When you enjoy an activity but never find the time to do it, your score will reflect this as a plus number times a minus one, resulting in a minus score. If you dislike something and never do it, this consistency will score as (-1) times (-1) which gives you a +1.

In order to complete your own satisfaction score, record your enjoyment responses and your frequency responses in the following table. For this computation we will list each response according to its weighted number. In the enjoyment chart, very much = 3, moderately = 2, some = 1, not at all = -1; on the frequency chart, daily = 3, weekly = 2, sometimes = 1, and never = -1. Please complete your responses by listing A and B scores and multiplying for each activity. Algebraic rules: plus times plus = plus; plus times minus = minus; minus times minus = plus. Thus, when you engage often in an activity you enjoy, you compute your score by multiplying a plus by a plus. When you enjoy an activity but never find the time to do it, your score will reflect this as a plus number times a minus one, resulting in a minus score. If you dislike something and never do it, this consistency scores as (-1) times (-1), which gives you a plus score.

After you have completed your satisfaction score, the next steps are obvious. Increase the frequency of those activities you truly enjoy. Re-structure your life so as to reduce the frequency of those activities you dislike, and increase your enjoyment of life.

Now is the time to practice happiness. Take time to enjoy life. Deliberately add pleasure to your days. Subtract from your life those activities which you do merely from habit, the dull routines which have long since ceased to give you pleasure. Subscribe to the principle of priority, and give first place in your energies to those activities which are truly enjoyable to you. If you like to fish, go fishing. If you enjoy playing bridge, make sure you do so. If you love art museums and hate hunting and fishing, the choices should be obvious. Forget about conventional stereotypes, and begin to enjoy your life. Do not use the preferences of your spouse or your friends as an excuse to avoid your own preferences. Maturity includes as a part of its parameters the ability to make decisions as individuals, and for each to allow the other freedom to function in that individuality. Cultivate those activities that bring you pleasure, and you will be rewarded by a sweetness of disposition which will enhance your relationships with those around you as well. Find what it takes to make you happy and make it your daily practice.

One of the keys to your happiness may turn out to be the same key that unlocks the door to continued prosperity. The list of people who have turned an avocation into an occupation is growing at an amazing rate. We met them everywhere we went, as you will.

Ross is one who turned a hobby into a business, and he literally got into it by the back door. Ross never had any idea that his habit of collecting junk would lead him into the commercial memorabilia business. Not that he calls it that. Ross collects old signs and old boxes because he likes them. He always has been fascinated with the way words can cause people to buy things.

Until five years ago Ross ran a combination general store and service station in a little town in Illinois at the crossroads of two state highways. He and Mabel managed a pretty good business for years. Ross was the second generation to make a living at the general store and collect signs on the side. His father, who started the business in the 1920's, had been a lot like Ross. He had never thrown anything away. When Ross came home from WWII he went into business with his father, and gradually they filled the big old barn in back of the store with signs and comic books and old boxes. The signs said everything from "His Master's Voice" to "Lucky Strike Green Has Gone to War" to "Lydia Pinkham." Mable did a little good natured grumbling, but Ross said it was the only thing the barn was used for anyway.

The town dwindled at about the same rate the barn filled. Some days Ross spent more time at estate sales than he did at the store. Still, he and Mable managed. They had a garden, raised a few chickens, visited with their neighbors, and held on.

Things changed dramatically five years ago when the new superhighway opened. Although the nearest exit ramp is only one mile away, Ross found out in a hurry that people will not ordinarily drive even one mile out of their way to buy gas. Ross was then fifty five—too young for social security, too old to move away and start over. While he and Mabel stewed in their limbo of worry, they went up to Chicago to visit their daughter. Mostly to take their mind off their problems, they went on a sight-seeing tour of Old Town. As Ross tells it, "When I looked at the junk they had decorating those fancy restaurants, I knew I had a gold mine out back in the barn."

Ross could hardly wait to get back home. He shut down the service station, invested some money in an eye catching interstate billboard that reads, "Commercial Memorabilia—Wholesale and Retail. Your cash for our Trash." He cleaned up the barn, displayed his favorite signs around in the stalls, put

Mable and the cash register in the wagon shed, and went into business. He was right. It has been a gold mine.

Many people have made challenge and change fit right into their happiness patterns. When Bill Lunt retired from his position as a sales executive, he decided to go public with his fifty year love affair with jazz. Bill has an encyclopedic knowledge of jazz that many a musicologist might envy, and an impressive record and tape collection. He now has his own radio program, and Bill's Big Band Sound airs on an affiliate station of National Public Radio. Dishing up an irresistible mix of fine jazz and wit and style, the program is enormously popular.

The implications for your own retirement are obvious. Study your own enjoyment chart, come to terms with what it takes to make you happy, and translate it into action.

If you were to meet Jim Trotter in connection with his summer job as a forest ranger in Estes National Park, Colorado, you would like him immediately. You would appreciate his confidence, be assured by his trustworthiness and be put at ease by his genuine liking for people. All these qualities enhance his job as a forest ranger, but Jim did not develop these characteristics solely in the forest. For the past forty years he has been a banker, realtor, and financial expert. The same character traits that are so desirable in a forest ranger are traits that have stood him in good stead through a rewarding career.

If you were to meet Jim and his wife, Betty, in their spacious home, rather than in the park, you would probably pick fairly standard adjectives to describe them: comfortable, conventional, kind, American as apple pie. They warrant all of these words, but there are others that apply. If you could catch a glimpse of Jim as he stands in front of a bazaar in India, discussing the future of the work of his church and its influence on the people of India, you would catch yet another vision. In India, he is an exuberant and evangelical executive.

Jim has turned his two major avocations into two quite different vocations. He and Betty and their sons have camped most summers for the past forty years, and his forest ranger duties are a happy extension of his hobby. His second vocation, his work for his church, enriches his life beyond the telling.

Jim began his ranger experience in 1945 as a college student on the G.I. Bill. Jim decided then that the only way he could afford a summer vacation was to combine both fun and profit. He sought and obtained employment that year as a ranger assigned to Mt. Lassen, California. The next summer he worked at Mt. Ranier. Jim has always remembered vividly the enjoyment of those summers. Last year, when he and Betty retired, they filled out applications with the National Park Service, and were thrilled that Jim was accepted.

Jim's assignments at Estes Park are to do whatever needs doing. He makes reservations, sells permits, answers questions, directs traffic, matches lost youngsters to worried parents, and does what he can for the tourists who come to the park to appreciate its beauties. Overall, his goal is to help preserve this beauty for future generations.

During the rest of the year Jim pursues his other career, acting as a roving ambassador for his church. His responsibilities for evangelical work in India have taken him on six trips to that fascinating and enigmatic country. He works there as an administrator and a problem solver. As an administrator, he brings encouragement, structure, hope, and discipline. His goal is to bring spiritual uplift to the evangelists stationed in India and to the thousands to whom they bring their message. Jim's duties as an elder in his church take up at least half of his time. As he assesses it now, he feels his retirement was essential. He had to retire in order to do the really important things in his life.

CHAPTER 16
ADD LIFE TO YOUR YEARS

"Gladness of the heart is the life of a man, and the joyfulness of a man prolongeth his days." Apocrypha

You know them when you see them. Easily recognized by their clear eyes, their firm skin, their trim bodies, they have the look of having struck a zestful bargain with life. We saw hundreds of them on the occasion of the first U.S. National Senior Olympics. Crowds of these remarkable people gathered to compete in athletic contests for persons 55 and over. The motivation of each contestant was the perennial challenge of physical competition. The goal of the planning committee was to set an image of seniors as fit and happy and able. We thought the event was a total success.

As remarkable for their attractive personalities as for their physical attractiveness, the more than 2,500 contestants gave overwhelming evidence of the positive linkage of mind and body. These are people accustomed to exertion and acquainted with sweat. They know how to translate fun and games into the rewards of winning.

Can winning make seniors happy and healthy and wise? We would argue that it can and it does. We saw zestful people, livelier, happier, and handsomer than could be imagined by their sedentary brothers and sisters. Most were more interested in competing with themselves than with the multitudes. For each one, the challenge of being his own best self was the contest that mattered the most, and a common thread ran through the stories. Each had improved his life and gladdened his heart through the daily discipline of physical exertion. These people have learned to put life in their years. Their days are marked by a sparkling and revitalizing energy.

Life's river is the sum of all its tributaries, both mental and physical. The tributaries determine whether the main stream is swift or sluggish. Just as streams either pollute or purify the river into which they flow, so do the influences that we let flow into our lives. A stagnant pool becomes fetid and unpleasant as it gradually dries up; a life without zest in a body without energy will eventually atrophy.

When we channel each tributary in terms of its positive effect, the results become a series of victories. When the bright stream of enthusiasm is predominant, it enriches every environment through which it passes. Independent of the restrictions of age, a remarkable woman has recently set a world record through her enthusiasm and accomplishments.

News stories recently described the philosophy of the 91-year old mountaineer who became the oldest woman to climb Japan's highest peak, Mt. Fuji. "You always feel good when you've made a goal," she said after her difficult three day climb. "You need goals!" Hulda Crooks began climbing at the age of 40. Her ascent of the 12,385 foot Mt. Fuji broke a record set in 1985 by a ninety year old. Hulda climbs for the challenge, and for the fun of the climb, but also to encourage other people to reject the limitations of age. She is conclusive proof that age is a state of mind.

You, too, can choose whether you will be young at 90 or old at thirty. It depends on whether you admit to the streams of your mind and your body the energizing tributaries that will keep you young. The discipline of daily physical exertion is remarkable medicine.

Louise believes that physical discipline can even lead to unexpected benefits to the character. When she hiked the Waterton/Glacier National Park a few years ago she found that her basic cowardice gave way to unsuspected gumption. Never notable for physical bravery, and handicapped by a fear of heights, Louise set out in the summer of her 59th year on a hiking expedition that changed her life. Intrigued by a seductive brochure, she made inadequate preparation for her journey. In the newspaper column she wrote for the *Cedar Rapids Gazette*, she described her adventure:

This is the story of a converted coward. Though bravery is not and never will be my strong point, I have just returned from a trip where I hiked in Waterton/Glacier National Park with the Smithsonian Associates. I will never be the same again. You might say that I have had a mountain-top experience.

My fear of heights was once so bad that walking right up to the glass windows to see the view from the Sears Tower in Chicago demanded a conscious act of will. Riding steep subway escalators used to be a white-knuckled, hand-gripping trip. Until very recently, I believed physical cowardice to be socially acceptable. But now that I've been through a wringer of an experience, I know better.

My planning for the hiking experience began with brochure-readings. I have always been gullible about the written word. When I signed on for this tour I was beguiled by selectively seductive prose that went something like this: "Hike through Alpine meadows and wooded forests. See breathtaking views of Glacier's magnificent peaks. Overnight in selected lodges and hotels."

Now, I envisioned all this accomplished while looking from the valley up to see the breathtaking views. Never in imagination's wildest streaks did I envision seeing these breathtaking views from the peaks down. I knew I would need stamina. I didn't know I would have to have courage, too. In retrospect, I presume I thought there would be 10 days of relatively sturdy hiking through gently sloping meadows of edelweiss, the snow-covered peaks in the background reverberating to melodic songs from "The Sound of Music."

As it turned out, wishing did not make it so. If there was a gentle slope, we didn't stay on it long enough make a joyful noise. The sounds I made were yelps and moans and never yodels. But the views were absolutely magnificent. These more than adequately compensated for my pain. In short, due to circumstances that rapidly got beyond my control, my cowardice rating dropped from a near-perfect 9.5 to a below-average 3 or 4.

This pilgrim's progress was so rapid that had the tour lasted longer I would have come back a callus-footed, strong-backed, insufferably smug mountain hiking expert. But even in the blister-footed, tired back and over-awed stage of a tenderfoot, a major transformation took place in me. I believe I have been irrevocably changed. No doubt this for the better. I am still a coward, but I am an improved coward.

I should have known when I met the cast of characters that I had gotten beyond my depth. It is hard to tell from first impressions how tough people really are, though I did get intimations of imperturbability. When we put on our hiking clothes and set out for the bus that would take us to Waterton National Park, I began to sense the mood of the pack I would be running with.

My hiking clothes had come from one of Iowa's better thrift shops. I got the whole set for $12.50 and felt fairly proud of myself for doing it, since I figured a well worn set of pants and shirts would work just as well if they had been broken in by someone else. So I set out in my baggy formerly worn pants and sweaters. My back-pack was new. My boots were in pretty good shape. But when I looked at my Smithsonian associates, it was clear that most if not all had been outfitted by L.L. Bean. Most were wearing things that had a well-worn look of good sturdy use on the trail. All at once I tumbled to the fact that these people had broken in their own trailclothes.

Their ages ranged from 22 to 72, and I immediately surmised that the 72-year-old would outhike me. I was equally sure the 22-year-old would lead the pack. Both assumptions were soon verified. At least half the group had the well formed leg muscles that testify to hours and hours of hiking. I was enormously cheered by seeing three or four associates whose L.L. Bean togs were brand new and whose muscles looked a tad shaky. I figured that I would have real competition for the dubious honor of finishing at the bottom of the hike. That turned out to be all too true.

The first day was fairly easy. We put our lunch packs in our backpacks and started up to see Bertha Lake, a five-mile hike, round-trip. The scenery was incredibly lovely. I didn't get out of breath more than ten times as we went up the first two and a half miles. I finished third from the bottom of a hiking string of 28 people.

By the second day, I had gained a bit more apprehension and a little more respect for high mountain air. The scenery continued to be incredibly gorgeous. I put on my old sloppy clothes, swung my leaking canteen around my shoulder and read the day's itinerary: "Round trip hike of 10 miles will take us to Crypt Lake and return." I couldn't imagine why a lake would be named Crypt Lake. Before the day was over I had the answer.

We started in an Alpine meadow, and I felt really good. We moved from there to forested slopes. I still felt good. By 11 a.m. we had gone beyond the forested slopes, and I had to pause often to rest on the switchbacks. As fellow travelers passed by, I heard snatches of conversation about how far it was to the ladder and the tunnel. Never having known before about the ladder and the tunnel, I began to ask apprehensive questions of each pilgrim who passed me by. Finally one said, "We do have to go up a ladder on this next cliff." That bit of scuttlebutt proved to be absolutely true.

I forced myself to look at the sheer granite face of a mountain, and there was the ladder. A mere ten feet in height, it might as well have been a hundred. Clearly, I was expected to climb up. I was not adverse to climbing up, though instantly I had the wit to forecast that I was apt to go into a fear-struck freeze when I had to climb down. Nevertheless, with some prodding from people behind me, and minor jeering from the people in front, I did inch my way up that ladder.

Immediately to the ladder's right was the entrance to a natural tunnel, in length about thirty feet. Since it was impossible to stand, obviously one had to crawl through. Other people seemed to be hit by claustrophobic fear at the tunnel entrance. Not me. I rejoiced to see it. When the rock hemmed me in, it was the only time the whole day I felt totally secure. With reluctance I left its safety and crawled through to the crypt's other side.

There in front of me loomed the worst part of the trip. To my right was a sheer drop. Directly in front was a narrow path. To my left was a steel cable placed in the granite cliff to be used by the cowards. Unfortunately, the cable had been placed at a height for an average man. At five-foot-three, I had a hard time grabbing onto it. Nevertheless, let me tell you, I managed.

It was at this point that the first of several appropriate verses of Scripture began to echo through my mind. As I grasped that steel cable and avoided looking down the mountain, the litany began: "Pride goeth before a fall." Since I know my pride was already gone, I prayed desperately that I could hang on and thereby avoid the fall. After an interminable interval, I did emerge on a rugged but wider path, and progressed on up to a most gorgeously beautiful lake.

There in a valley was Crypt Lake, set like a jewel among snow-clad peaks. I sat there, dipped my feet in its glacier-fed waters and tried to eat lunch. My stomach rebelled. That cowardly stomach knew it would have to go back down the same trail it had come up. Privately, I renamed Crypt Lake as the

Valley of Humiliation. All too soon it was time to go back. I'll spare you the return trip's details. Nothing ever was that bad again. Absolutely, nothing in the whole trip ever came close to the experience of going down that ladder.

On the third day we hiked to the rim of the world. I set out in fine fettle, having soaked away most of my aches, both psychic and physical. My lungs adjusted to the altitude; my surroundings adjusted my attitude. I made it to the top without major mishap. It was as I sat there eating lunch, looking all the way around at the peaks, valleys, lakes, and meadows that comprised an awe-inspiring view, that I was born again. I realized the view and sense of wonder and inspiration were worth it all.

And there, sitting on that five foot wide flat rock, looking 360 degrees around the slopes of this incredible mountain, I decided I was sitting in the center of the whole wide world. Obviously God had made the view to improve the character of foot-sore pilgrims.

From that day on, pride and fun took over. I won't say my strength got drastically improved, but it got considerably improved. I moved up from the position of third from the last to just short of the middle of the group, and there I stayed. I took real pride in being able to tough out the day. There is a feeling of inspiration and joy that comes from seeing nature at its incredible best. My fellow travelers had their own set of peak experiences, and it was with a fine sense of esprit de corps that we managed each morning to thrust our beat-up feet back into our well worn boots and start out again to see what God hath wrought.

I began to experience that marvelous feeling that comes from concentrating only on the here and now, the moment itself. All my usual concerns, all my petty peeves and gripes faded into nothing as I contemplated how best to place my feet so as to hike across a snowbank without sliding 200 feet down the slope.

Events of the last day provided a fitting climax to all that had gone before. We were scheduled to hike down from Granite Park Chalet, a rustic lodge located near the continental divide. The weather appeared threatening. We were informed by the Park Service that we had approximately five hours in which to hike out, as it was expected that the trail would soon be closed by snow.

That easy downhill final hike got extremely complicated by the blizzard that developed, but even here there were compensations. We came to a large snowfield on which six big-horned rams were tentatively contesting for leadership. As we stood there, fascinated, no more than 100 feet from these rams, it was as though we were on another planet. I couldn't have felt farther from Cedar Rapids, Iowa, had I been at that moment standing on the edge of a crater on the moon.

With real reluctance, we left the rams and continued our forced march through the snow. The last pass of the day was, to say the least, memorable. The Park Service had very thoughtfully set another one of those steel cables along the side of the mountain, thereby helping me through another heart-thumping experience. Hiking a trail along a sheer drop in dry weather is one thing. What I had done seven days before now looked to be kid stuff compared to hiking a similar trail covered with slippery snow. I blessed our Park Service, and I clutched onto that cable until I soaked my mittens, and blistered my hands.

As we emerged at the trailhead on the highway,

forest rangers gathered us into their bus and deposited a cold, wet, hungry, yet triumphant little bunch of returning pilgrims in the lobby of a really fine resort hotel. We must have been the most disheveled, wretched-looking guests the place ever received.

Yet I experienced that feeling of elation which comes from having tackled and toughed out something really difficult. At that moment, despite my tired and miserable condition, I wouldn't have changed places with any one of those superior-looking people who stared at us as we trudged across the hotel lobby.

Louise concluded, "Being born again is not easy, but I can hardly wait for another chance for a revival experience."

What experiences have you planned for your freedom third? What fantasies of your youth are with you still?

The current life expectancies of Americans over fifty would have amazed our ancestors, and science continues to discover ways to prolong our lives even further. The average sixty year old in America can expect another eighteen years. But the general population statistics obscure the possibility that you may well live to be a hundred. If the current pattern of longevity continues, by the year 2000 it is estimated that there will be 100,000 people over one hundred in America. The challenge for each of us is to live these years with the imagination of a child, the discipline of an adult and the eagerness of an adolescent.

Ashley Montague, in his book, *Growing Young*, lists twenty six traits of a child, traits which he believes must be retained by those who would stay young at heart: love, friendship, sensitivity; the need to think soundly; the need to know, to learn, to work, to organize; curiosity; wonder; playfulness; imagination, creativity; open-mindedness; flexibility, experimental-mindedness; the willingness to explore; resiliency; humor; joy; laughter and tears; optimism; honesty and trust; compassionate intelligence; dance; and song. These are the tributaries which, if allowed to flow through the river of your life, can cause it to sparkle with a clear beauty and retain a delicious freshness. The mythology of old age is misleading. Those whose spirits remain eternally youthful can testify that there are times when the heart leaps in happiness. In defiance of chronological age, we then feel delightfully, ridiculously, young.

Release yourself from the tyranny of convention. The tyranny of the opinion of others restrains courage and inhibits delight. In truth, becoming your own best self—cultivating your own special qualities—is sometimes neither admired nor encouraged. Do not let this deter you.

Even though the body grows old, the spirit need not grow old with it.

Flexibility diminishes when the body is sedentary, and youthfulness of spirit is diminished by a sedentary mind. Those who keep physically limber and intellectually stimulated can give the lie to the myth of old age. The myth that a second childhood is equivalent to senility is a narrow and callous view. The deliberate cultivation of the joys of childhood can influence our lives with an enthusiasm that can revitalize our world. A renaissance fueled by the contributions of the elderly could be a renaissance informed by wisdom and defined by compassion.

There are certain unacceptable losses: a curiosity

about life, the ability to have fun, the ability to laugh, an eagerness to learn. These are as necessary to the agility of the mind and the spirit as physical exercise is to the agility of the body. Will you give yourself the freedom to be young at heart? Will you give yourself the freedom to be yourself?

CHAPTER 17
THE
DIPLOMA—HAPPINESS

"The heart of a man changeth his countenance, whether it be for good or evil." The Holy Bible: Apocrypha

We humbly offer the following six rules as curriculum requirements for the most important degree of all, the diploma in the art of living. We believe that the formula for happiness has six parts:
1. Remember your roots.
2. Live in your present.
3. Cherish your friends.
4. Make use of your talents.
5. Acknowledge your dreams.
6. Live in harmony with your heart.

The mystery of happiness is that those who seek it as such never find it. Happiness is not a destination, not a goal; happiness comes from within. There is a formula which describes it. It is written in the ink of service and translated through the language of love. Happiness is really only a by-product of doing for others. Many spend their lives unhappily searching for that which is within their reach, not realizing that happiness is a treasure not to be found from without but from within.

Cavett believes that there is a lowest common denominator for happiness, and that this lowest common denominator forms the basis for all the parts of our formula. This denominator is service to others, one of life's greatest gifts is the ability to take inventory of ourselves and rededicate our lives to the art of living. From his vantage point of almost eighty years, Cavett has evolved his own philosophy. He believes that if a person truly loves others and feels a deep need to serve them, happiness will take on the dimension of blessedness. On the other hand, he has observed that the rewards of this life have a way of eluding those who are seduced by selfishness and who put self-interest above that of the capacity to consider others.

All of us know that Thomas Jefferson was one of the giants of history. Not many realize that he was also one of the happiest and most personable men in Virginia. Students of his life have made it clear that he truly enjoyed serving. Jefferson's epitaph, which he wrote himself, is more noted for the things omitted that for those contained. This great man died on the fiftieth anniversary of American independence. His epitaph reads:

"Here was buried Thomas Jefferson, author of the Declaration of Independence, of the Statute of Virginia for Religious Freedom, and Father of the University of Virginia."

Jefferson's daughter was asked why there were not included the facts that he had been governor of Virginia, minister to France, secretary of state, and president of the United States. She explained that her father in answer to this same question, had replied, "The things which are not on my inscription are things people did for me. The things that are on it are things I did for the people."

With the knowledge that all the different parts of our formula are based on our relationships with the world around us, let us now consider each:

1. *Remember your roots.* In Louise's little home town in Arkansas there is an annual rite of convergence. They call it Homecoming, and hold it the first Sunday in June.

Begun in the summer of 1930 when the country was in the grip of a terrible depression, Homecoming was designed to provide a counteracting expression of strength and hope. Hundreds of invitations were mailed out on penny postcards to friends and relatives who had formerly lived there. Both the residents and those natives who had moved away needed all the hope they could get that summer.

So persuasive were the invitations that a record crowd assembled. Their optimism shaken but not destroyed by the worst drought in memory, folks began their three-day weekend with music and visiting and carrying on. On Saturday the rain began—a long, soaking, crop-saving rain. Spirits ran so high that the crowd at the Sunday service overflowed the church and filled the church yard.

After nearly sixty years, things have changed some. But for those who no longer live there, the familiar ritual of seeking out their earliest memories has not lessened in its pleasure. Undeniably, the cast of characters has changed, as all the roles have been handed down a generation or two. Then, too, a bit of affluence has finally made itself felt, even in Arkansas.

An efficient super highway splits the state through the middle now. The county seat boasts a pleasant motel adjacent to the crowded highway. Annually,

Louise and her brother and sister meet there, along with as many of their children as can be persuaded to join them for this sentimental journey. After they check in and clean up, they head through the hills for home.

As Louise tells the story: "The road to our town is paved now. We think it is a big improvement over the grit and gravel of our childhood. The trip that used to take an hour speeds by in twenty minutes. From the time we cross the clear creek and crest the high hill on its far bank, we know we're home again. Our first glimpse of the large and lovely reach of the sheltering Boston Mountains reminds us that this was our first standard of panoramic beauty. We remark again about the view, as awed as though we hadn't seen it every day for the first several years of our lives.

"There are differences, of course. The grass is greener, the sky is bluer, the mountains are larger, our homeplace is smaller, the church is dearer, and the cemetery is fuller. We go to the cemetery first, and note with gentle approval that our parents lie surrounded by friends, their graves grouped as gregariously as were their lives.

"Next, we drive to the town square and gear up for the festivities. Hugging old friends, tenderly kissing the cheeks of our more ancient relatives, we thoroughly enjoy the touches of sentiment. Throughout the evening and continuing on past the church rituals the next morning, we indulge in remembrances, enlarging the best, conveniently forgetting the worst.

When we say good-bye and begin our journeys to our present homes, we are high on our own Ozarkian brand of emotional champagne. We find it infinitely more satisfying than the liquid kind."

Although Louise has not lived in Arkansas since she was eighteen, so deep are her roots that it was many years before she would even acknowledge other places as home. Many decades later, she now knows that most of us find more than one home in our lives.

Roots are essential, for they define our lives. We ignore them at our peril, but, important as they are, they are no substitute for new growth. Our second rule, then, is even more important than the first.

2. *Live in your Present*. Appreciate this moment, for it is reality. The remembrance of things past may be a fragrance or an odor, but it is only a wafting on the breezes of the memory, not the substantial reality of the here and now. Each day brings the chance once more to weave a new pattern into the fabric of your life. Look on this chance as the miracle it is.

Discipline yourself to live your days as twenty four hour compartments, and enjoy each one like a jewel. When we come to terms with that inner knowledge that separates us from the other animals, the knowledge that our days are numbered, it puts our lives in sharp focus. The simplest comforts become pleasures, the world around us reveals its beauty, and the affection of those we love becomes even more precious. The miracle of a longer life span, the opportunity to enjoy life through decades denied to our ancestors—these are blessings which deserve our deepest gratitude. We are the first generation in the history of mankind to have such an extended lifespan. Surely we will want to use this opportunity well, and to live each day as the treasure it is. Our generation has been granted an unprecedented gift.

If you will remind yourself each morning that this is the only time you will live this particular day it will set an enthusiastic mood for the daily adventure of life. Start your day in an expectant frame of mind. Avoid pessimism and avoid the pessimistic.

Cavett tells the story of a pessimistic man whose attitude could best be described as an accident waiting to happen. This particular man was sitting in a restaurant in Dallas, Texas, smoking a large cigar, and reading the newspaper between gulps of food. A lovely and sparkling young waitress poured his coffee, and smilingly said, "It's a wonderful day, isn't it?" Without glancing up from his paper, the man growled through a mouthful of eggs and a half chewed cigar, "What's so wonderful about it?" The little waitress assessed him accurately and cheerfully, and in her southern drawl replied, "Mister, I tell you, you oughta try missin' a few and you'll find out!" Cavett swears that the man brightened up the whole room simply by walking out of it.

Translated into the positive, the formula for appreciation of the present is magically simple. Remember that today is the greatest day of your life until tomorrow. Life is as full as you will let it be.

3. *Cherish Your Friends.* Cleanliness may or may not be next to Godliness, but we are convinced that friendship is. Throughout the ages the stories of friendships have been told: David and Jonathan, Damon and Pythias, Darby and Joan. One of the sweetest stories in the Old Testament, that of Ruth and Naomi in the alien corn, was based on the love and friendship between mother-in-law and daughter-in-law, and not on the ties of blood. Scholars and philosophers have given us splendid descriptions of friendship:

"A friend is, as it were, a second self."

"The best mirror is an old friend."

"A friend may well be reckoned the masterpiece of nature."

We offer one of our own: "A friend knows you through and through and likes you anyway."

Friends understand us. Friends offer their company, comfort and compassion in the give and take of daily living. Friends rejoice with us and coach us on the journey to our triumphs. It is not difficult to find those who will weep with us in time of misfortune. Many will offer comfort during the miseries of life. Even acquaintances are excellent at commiseration.

Twenty five hundred years ago, Aeschyles observed that it is in the character of very few men to honor without envy a friend who has prospered. It takes a true friend to wish you well while you are winning, and to wish you joy from the bottom of a generous heart. Friends want us to be happy. Friends stand ready to help in the process. There are qualities which are mercifully absent from friendships...hypocrisy, deceit, pretense...and their absence leaves room for the lovely virtue of charity. Friends see us with that remarkable vision which simultaneously blurs our flaws and enlarges our strengths.

We need to cultivate our friends and cherish them as though they have inestimable value, as indeed they do. We often compare our friends to familiar objects. "She's as comfortable as an old shoe," we say of one well-loved and easy to be around. But friends are much more than serviceable companions and much more than familiar sources of comfort. Each friend represents a special part of the world as we know it, a world which would not be possible without this unique individual. The deep and particular knowledge which exists between true friends creates always a unique portion of our world.

Cicero's truth is with us still. He said, 'In nothing do we approach so nearly to the gods as doing good to men.'

4. *Make Use of Your Talents.* We who are the fortunate citizens of America have had a proud legacy handed down to us by leaders of the past. We have been taught that privilege and talent are to be repaid through service. The idle rich are considered to be apart from the best of American tradition. In our generation we are accustomed to working. And those retirees who work as volunteers seem to work as hard and as consciously as though they were being paid for it. As, of course, they are—paid in satisfaction of knowing that a necessary job is well done. Whether your work in your freedom third is rewarded in money, in satisfaction, or in a happy combination of both, the use of your true talents is one of the most satisfying ventures on this great planet.

The productive use of our talents translate directly into pride...pride in ourselves, pride in the accomplishments of our friends and neighbors, and finally, pride of place and country. Most of us are proud of doing whatever it is we have learned to do well. Whether you bake a cake, build a bridge, discover a drug, soothe a child, or carve a statue, to enjoy the doing and to do it well is one of life's true pleasures.

Bertrand Russell in his excellent book, the *Conquest of Happiness*, points out that some kinds of skilled work (he uses politics as an example) require so much wisdom that people are at their best between sixty and seventy. Such persons, he believed, are happier at age 70 than other persons of equal age. We would presume to expand on Mr. Russell's statement. The retirees we talked to who had designed tasks that matched their talents said they were happier than they had ever been in their lives. For these, the decades of their 60s and 70s and 80s were truly their golden years. These people, constructively filling their time according to their own choice, have progressed high on the ladder of civilization. Prolonged idleness brings boredom, but purposeful accomplishment, Russell tells us, is one of the most essential ingredients of happiness in the long run. It cures the habit of hatred, displaces envy, and brings enjoyment to our days. The satisfying use of our talents is not the whole of life, but it is a necessary part, and when combined with affection and appreciation it adds enormously to our capacity for zest.

5. *Acknowledge Your Dreams.* Nothing great in life was ever accomplished until it was born in the shape of a dream. As the oak sleeps in the acorn, so are our dreams the seedlings of reality. He was a scientist, Albert Einstein, who said "Imagination is more important than knowledge." Margaret Cousins tells us, "People cannot live without stories any more than they can live without bread." We are not advocating that you live exclusively in a dream world—far from it—but we do believe that when we cease to hope and dream and imagine our very spirits wither. We do not for one moment believe that those of us in our freedom third should feel that the time for dreams has passed us by. The dreams of our maturity have a quality that the dreams of our youth can never match. The dreams of youth are tempered by maturity. The education afforded by life can be summed up in the statement that education is what you have left

over after you subtract what you have forgotten from what you have learned. This difference is small in youth, grows considerably in adulthood, and looms large in maturity. And it is this difference which is the foundation of our most vital dreams.

Both Einstein and Edison were once regarded as hopeless dreamers. Yet they and all the great creators in our civilization first dreamed, then accomplished. There cannot be one without the other. When Jim Trotter is working for his church in India, he is building his dream with the lumber of reality. When Barbara works to design a system to improve education in this country, she is working from the blueprint of her dreams. The entrepreneur who is now in the beginning stages of owning his own business is responding to his long-time dream of being his own boss. Dreams are vital, for they inform reality.

Many believe that dreams have within themselves the power to generate all those qualities that make dreams come true. We must take care, therefore, to dream the right dreams, have the right visions, and desire the right things, for dreams do come true. They can lead to happiness or to miseries. The dreams of your youth, tempered by time and strengthened by wisdom, may be even better than the original vision.

What long held dream of yours is still waiting to be accomplished?

6. *Live in Harmony with your Heart.* How often have we heard it said about someone, "He can do the job, but his heart is not in it?" Such people are all too easy to find. You will see them dutifully going through the necessary motions—motions based on logical rules and learned behavior. Their actions are characterized by qualities absent as much as by qualities pres-

ent. The absence of zest and joy and spontaneity is balanced by the presence of structure and duty and resignation. Nature does, indeed, abhor a vacuum, but fills the space without mercy.

The price of disharmony is heavy. Over time, the practice of activities which emphasize the head at the expense of the heart will leave their mark: when duty consistently rules over desire, the marks are etched on the face. We have all heard the truism that happy people paint their faces from the inside. These are the wise and fortunate ones who have orchestrated a two-part harmony between their minds and their hearts. There is a loveliness which comes from this harmony, a loveliness unmistakably translated into the physical fetures of those so favored.

Conversely, the mean spirited acquire a pinched and rigid look; the unwilling are characterized by begrudging and unhappy countenance. Yet it need not be this way. Your own heart contains guides which are trustworthy. It is human nature to go eagerly to work that we love, and to prize the accomplishments earned as a result of these efforts. This congruency between what we do and what we like to do constitutes a real blessing.

We believe this blessing to be within the reach of all. The resolution of conflict between the heart and the will is the essential choice necessary for a happy life.

At the core of this choice is the need to come to terms with the hopes of your own heart. Long ago, a poet sang that the desire accomplished is sweet to the soul. We assure you that if you desire happiness you must harmonize your head and your heart. If you desire to become that person who is your own true self, and if you design your life in patterns faithful to this desire, you will be rewarded by success. And it will truly be sweet to your soul.

We all live by two sets of rules. One is the set designed by the outside world, and it is tremendously important. The wisdom of the ages has been transmitted through it. The other set of rules lives in your heart, and it is equally important. Please do not live the only life you have eternally trying to conform to the code of others, without coming to terms with the hopes of your own heart.

Wisdom is not bought, nor happiness borrowed. In association with enthusiasm and charity and joy, these blessings keep company with the hopes of your heart.

Life itself is such a gift that each day is precious in its own right. To walk in health on the face of this fragrant earth, to see its beauties and to hear its music is to know happiness. Sometimes, in the clear light of a bright morning, joy can actually be felt in the bones.

Life gets fragile and infinitely precious when reason tells us we have less ahead than we have behind. Treasure each day for the miracle it is. Live your life in gladness. Affirm your choice. You have chosen to live a good life and to live it more abundantly. Happiness consists of loving life.

The End

STAY HEALTHY WITH WARNER BOOKS!

___ **LIFE EXTENSION**   *(L38-735, $14.95, U.S.A.)*
A Practical Scientific   *($17.50, CAN)*
Approach
by Durk Pearson and Sandy Shaw

Durk Pearson and Sandy Shaw present a vital new science that can change the quality of your life. This exciting book explains how you can slow your own aging while improving your current health, mental abilities, controlling your weight, and more. No one can afford to overlook the revolutionary advances that are revealed in this ground-breaking new book.

___ **LIFE EXTENSION**   *(L38-560, $10.95, U.S.A.)*
COMPANION   *($11.95, CAN)*
by Durk Pearson and Sandy Shaw

Now the authors of the #1 bestseller **Life Extension** offer you a practical guide to personal health improvement. In easy-to-understand layman's language, here are the latest, up-to-the-minute findings on aging and vital information about vitamins, nutrients, and prescription drugs to help you solve common health problems without drastically changing your current lifestyle.

 Warner Books P.O. Box 690
New York, NY 10019

Please send me the books I have checked. I enclose a check or money order (not cash), plus 95¢ per order and 95¢ per copy to cover postage and handling.* (Allow 4-6 weeks for delivery.)

___Please send me your free mail order catalog. (If ordering only the catalog, include a large self-addressed, stamped envelope.)

Name _____

Address _____

City_____ State _____ Zip_____

*New York and California residents add applicable sales tax.

America's #1 Diet Book Experts!
HARVEY & MARILYN DIAMOND

☐ **FIT FOR LIFE**
(L30-015, $4.95, U.S.A.) (L30-016, $5.95, Canada)
Two-million-copy national bestseller!
The natural body cycle, permanent weight-loss plan that proves it's not only what you eat, but also when and how. The perfect solution for those who want to be at their best.

Also available:

☐ **FIT FOR LIFE II: LIVING HEALTH**
(L34-660, $4.95, U.S.A.) (L34-661, $5.95, Canada)
A whole new approach to total and permanent good health that shows you how everything around you is potentially valuable or harmful to your health.

**Warner Books P.O. Box 690
New York, NY 10019**

Please send me the books I have checked. I enclose a check or money order (not cash), plus 95¢ per order and 95¢ per copy to cover postage and handling.* (Allow 4-6 weeks for delivery.)

___Please send me your free mail order catalog. (If ordering only the catalog, include a large self-addressed, stamped envelope.)

Name _____

Address _____

City _____ State _____ Zip _____

*New York and California residents add applicable sales tax.